Holiday in Hell

Titles in Harvestime's **Winning Through** series:

Holiday in Hell — *A harrowing journey through M.E.,*
by Chris Youngman

Stigma! — *An AIDS widow's story,*
by Jo-Anne Cohrs

Love Me, Please! — *One woman's search for security,*
by Beverly Wells

Give Me Children! — *Why can't I be a mother?,*
by Margaret Howson

A companion video to this book, *They Claim a Miracle: The Chris Youngman Story,* has been produced by Dales Television and can be hired from leading video centres. In case of difficulty, or if you wish to purchase a copy, contact: Dales Television, Nettle Hill, Brinklow Road, Ansty, Coventry CV7 9JL, UK.

Holiday in Hell

A harrowing journey through M.E.

Chris Youngman

with Edwina Allison

Harvestime

Published in the United Kingdom by:
Harvestime Publishing Ltd, 69 Main Street, Markfield
Leicester LE6 0UT

Copyright © 1988 Chris Youngman & Edwina Allison
First published by Harvestime
First printed November 1988
Reprinted January 1991

British Library Cataloguing in Publication Data

Youngman, Chris
Holiday in hell. — (Winning through).
1. Myalgic encephalomyelitis victims.
Personal observations.
I. Title II. Allison, Edwina III. Series
ISBN 0-947714-64-2

Printed and bound in the United Kingdom by:
Richard Clay Ltd, Bungay, Suffolk

Contents

Dedication

With our grateful love to Joy and Derek Tyler, who had the answer, and with affection and thanks to all the medical staff who helped and supported us, especially my general practitioner and the two consultants

1

The nightmare begins

It was a beautiful punchbowl. Round, deep, with eight funny little cups hanging around its sides. I picked it up to have a closer look, marvelling at its weight, running my hands over the smooth yellow-ochre clay.

I turned to my husband, Peter. I knew what he'd be thinking: 'Where on earth are we going to put it?' Our car, a battered blue Citroen, was parked on the hill outside the pottery, packed to capacity and swamped by an enormous bundle of camping gear which perched, like a monstrous growth, on its back.

Sally, our daughter, had to sit squashed in the back seat surrounded by pots and pans, food and mountains of bedding. It would be a miracle if we could fit in one more thing.

'Oh, let's buy it!' he said recklessly, having fallen in love with it too.

But I couldn't answer him. He stared at me, his smile fading as he took in my ashen face and blue lips. My head was spinning, the room reeling drunkenly around me. Peter, Sally and shelves of pottery all seemed to rush towards me before falling away, disappearing into muffled blackness.

Suddenly conscious of the punchbowl still in my hands,

I gathered together all my powers of concentration and carefully set it down again. 'I feel rotten,' I gasped. 'I'm going to sit in the car.'

On jelly-like legs I made my way across the pottery, out of the door to the waiting car and sank gratefully into the passenger seat. Wave after wave of illness swept over me; an icy numbness spread through my body, chilling me to the bone.

Peter and Sally arrived, triumphantly bearing the precious punchbowl they had stayed to pay for.

'Feeling better now?' they asked casually. I shook my head.

'You'll be all right in a few minutes,' said Peter reassuringly, starting up the car. 'You're probably exhausted after helping to pack up the wet tent this morning.'

I wasn't convinced. This didn't feel like mere tiredness. It was more like flu or some other nasty bug.

'What a time to be ill,' I thought miserably. We were camping in the middle of France. Peter couldn't speak a word of the language. What were we going to do? I knew one thing. I couldn't face camping while I felt like this. I closed my eyes and lay back in my seat, utterly wretched.

The car slowed to a halt. I opened my eyes and saw we were parked in a layby.

'Chris—are you all right? You look awful!' Peter took hold of my icy hand. 'You're frozen. You're shivering!' he exclaimed.

He got out of the car and began unpacking the camping

gear. I felt too weak to even ask what he was doing. A few minutes later he came back with a hot-water bottle, lovingly made on the Camping Gaz stove by the side of the road.

'You need to be in bed, love,' he said gently. 'I'm going to take you to Lucille's.'

Lucille! Of course! A mixture of relief and dismay rose up within me.

Our friend Lucille lived in northern France. We'd stayed with her for a couple of days when we first arrived and she had given us a spare key to her house so that we could call again to break our journey on the way home. She'd had to go away but we knew she wouldn't mind if we stayed there until I felt better.

The trouble was, Lucille lived in Amiens—almost a hundred miles away. It would take ages to get there and would completely mess up our holiday plans.

But I felt too ill to care. I huddled in my seat clutching the hot-water bottle, which made no impression on the paralysing cold which by now had gripped my body, shaking me from head to toe.

The decision made, we began to retrace the route which had brought us to our campsite just outside Paris. On and on we drove. The car, which had eaten up the miles so easily before, now seemed to crawl along. Gradually the journey assumed a nightmarish quality, grotesquely blurred by nausea and the pain in my back and head.

It was impossible to believe that we had travelled those same roads in the opposite direction laughing and chattering. Our washing, pegged out to dry like gaily-coloured bunting across the struts of the sunroof opening, had caused great merriment among our fellow-holidaymakers as they overtook us on the broad, tree-lined avenues.

Amiens. At last we arrived in Lucille's home-town. It was late, and we dropped thankfully into bed, exhausted. But I couldn't sleep. The pain was so excruciating that no matter how I lay I couldn't get comfortable. A strong suspicion gripped my mind. Meningitis! Suppose I had meningitis?

I worked as senior physiotherapist, running a rehabilitation unit at our local hospital, so I knew about meningitis. If I were taken into hospital they would almost certainly perform tests to confirm such a diagnosis. One of them involved putting a needle into the spine to draw off some of the fluid there. I couldn't face undergoing such tests in a foreign country. My French wasn't fluent enough for me to cope.

'I'm *not* going to hospital,' I thought fiercely. 'I know I'll be all right if I can just rest for a while.'

A week went by, but still I didn't feel any better. Sitting up was such a struggle that I had to gulp two or three mouthfuls of food then collapse, exhausted, on to the pillows again.

Reaching the bathroom, situated along the landing and down a short flight of stairs, demanded a Herculean effort. Too dizzy to risk walking downstairs, I would crawl on hands and knees there and back.

Towards the end of the week Sally said anxiously, 'I'm worried about Lucille's little budgie, Mum.' I had to laugh.

Here I was, feeling terribly ill, yet my thirteen-year-old daughter was worrying about a budgerigar!

I tottered shakily across the room to investigate. The poor thing certainly looked pathetic—in fact, it looked pretty much as I felt!

'What's the matter, little pet? What's wrong?' I crooned to it sympathetically.

'It lost its mate recently,' Peter explained.

A picture of abject misery, the little creature sat huddled on its perch, love-lorn and bereaved. Despite my own misery my heart went out to it. We decided to buy it another mate. 'But not one that's too posh,' I advised, as Peter and Sally went out to the pet shop. 'Try to find one it will feel comfortable with.'

They returned, giggling at the French pet-shop owner's reaction to these mad English customers who had insisted on buying the most bedraggled budgie in the aviary.

I was right. Far from feeling threatened by the new arrival, the little bird rushed up and down on his perch, ringing his bell in delight. They snuggled up together like two lovebirds. That is one of the few happy memories we have of our holiday.

Lucille came back home and, with her to act as interpreter, I felt safe to visit the doctor. Although still very weak, I was able to sit up long enough to make the journey.

'The doctor says you have a virus infection,' explained Lucille. 'You mustn't think of travelling home until you're much better.'

It was embarrassing. How dreadful for her to be put

upon by three uninvited guests, one drooping around the house like a sickly ghost, the other two anxious and irritated, waiting for her to get better! But Lucille made us very welcome and did everything possible to make us comfortable.

'Oh, what a waste of our holiday,' I thought guiltily. I tried to act and speak normally, pretending that I felt better but having to summon up all my will power just to stay on my feet. We even had an outing to a cavern, but what should have been a happy sightseeing day was for me a nightmare to be endured.

'Please take me home, Peter,' I begged miserably. 'It isn't fair to put upon Lucille any longer.'

'The doctor says you can't go home until you're much better,' he insisted.

'I am, I am,' I lied, desperately.

Acutely aware that Lucille's two young daughters were in exile at a relative's house in case my illness was infectious, he finally agreed. 'But only halfway,' he decided. 'We'll stay with my mother to break the journey so that you can rest a while.'

So, waving goodbye to a relieved Lucille, we set off for England and arrived at Mother's home in Essex in glorious sunshine.

She was kindness itself, gently tucking me into bed and fussing over Sally and Peter, giving them a chance to rest, too, after caring for me for the past fortnight.

I lay staring up at the ceiling, in Peter's old bed, in the room he had occupied before we were married. Out in the sunny garden he sat chatting with Sally. I listened to them and thought of all the plans we'd made for our holiday. All the things we'd intended to do. The places we should have visited.

'What a rotten holiday,' I thought, bitterly. It was all my fault. I'd ruined everything.

If I'd known what was to come, that would have been the least of my worries.

2

A military operation

I could hardly believe this was happening to me. Me! Lying around the house, barely able to sit up long enough to eat!

People who knew me marvelled at the amount of energy I usually had. I was always so healthy, so full of life. I not only held down a demanding job as a physiotherapist, but I led keep-fit classes, too.

And now the responsibility of these jobs, which I had so enjoyed, was weighing heavily upon me. So many people were being inconvenienced by my absence that I felt I must get better quickly for their sake.

As soon as we got home from Essex I saw my family doctor and described to him the mysterious illness which had doomed our holiday to failure. He sent me to the local hospital for blood tests and prescribed a week's bed-rest.

I knew that the result of my enforced idleness would be chaos unless I organised those who were dependent on me with all the precision of a general planning a military operation.

The phone never stopped ringing. First it would be my colleague, Susan, asking advice about the treatment of a patient. Next, a member of the keep-fit class would want details of when our class would be starting again after the long summer break. How could I tell her that her teacher was too unfit even to stagger downstairs to answer the phone? We fixed for one to be fitted by the bed so I could lie there and deal with its constant ringing.

To add to my difficulties, reporters from the local newspapers were ringing to make arrangements to interview me about my forthcoming art exhibition, and asking when photographs could be taken. It was only a small local exhibition but still very important to us as it was being held to publicise the opening of a friend's shop.

Also, our family holidays were financed by the sale of my paintings. Wildlife and flowers were my specialities, and I was developing a new style using wax and inks. My latest venture was painting cat pictures for a shop in Covent Garden, London. This illness was messing up every area of my life.

'Why aren't I getting any better?' I wondered impatiently. I felt so weary! And it wasn't an ordinary tiredness—deep down I felt completely exhausted. And I was due to return to work the next day.

I ran a small rehabilitation unit at a crumbling old hospital which had been converted, long ago, from a Victorian workhouse. The buildings, crowned with pigeons and entwined with a network of steaming, creaking pipes, were due to be demolished shortly. But for the moment the little room above the boiler house played a major role in retraining people who had suffered physical brain damage.

Brought from hospital wards by ambulance, or helped by friends and relatives, they came to relearn the everyday skills which we all take for granted and which they were now bewilderingly unable to perform. Walking, dressing, eating; some no longer able to speak but forced to communicate in a series of undignified grunts and signs, each one a victim of a hitherto undreamt-of disaster.

It was hard work for all of us, and called for every ounce of skill and patience I possessed—but I loved it. That little physiotherapy unit was my life.

The next morning I could hardly crawl out of bed and into the car to get to work on time. I've never been too lively first thing, but this was different! I arrived at the hospital, changed into my uniform and, after a much-needed cup of coffee, made my way across the grounds to the unit which was my own domain.

No patients yet. That was a relief. Everything looked exactly the same as it had before I went away. The long Formica-topped tables down the centre of the room; the enormous red geriatric chair in the bay window by the phone; the dining chairs pushed together into one corner.

I went to move them into position around the tables so that everything would be ready when the ambulance arrived with its first cargo of patients. I couldn't lift them!

'What's the matter with me?' I thought, irritated by my own weakness. It was ridiculous. The chairs weren't particularly heavy—I was used to swinging them around easily. Puzzled and discouraged, I sat and waited for the rest of the staff to arrive to do it for me.

'Hello! Welcome back,' called Rita, my assistant,

coming from the room upstairs. 'Did you have a good holiday?'

I watched as she hastily arranged the chairs around the table, not even seeming to notice their weight. Then the doors swung open and the first patients arrived.

It quickly became obvious that I couldn't cope with my normal working routine. The patients, distressed at seeing their usually bouncing physio feeble and exhausted, rallied round magnificently, the fitter ones helping the less mobile, fetching and carrying for them.

'You sit down, Mrs Youngman. We'll do the exercises by ourselves today; we know the routine,' they said kindly. So I collapsed into the geriatric high-seated chair, unable to do anything more active than offer advice and answer the phone.

'What a relief that's over,' I thought, driving out of the hospital carpark. I longed to get home and lie down. My head felt muzzy, my hands and legs weak.

Then, suddenly, all strength disappeared from my hands and feet. I couldn't steer the wheel or press the pedals; my body refused to respond. I simply couldn't believe it! The car rolled slowly to a halt by the side of the road and I sat, my hands limply draped across the steering-wheel, wondering what on earth to do.

Gradually, strength returned and I felt able to carry on. Like a learner driver on her first lesson, I cautiously eased the car into gear and crept off along the road. I had to pass my doctor's surgery on the way home, so I decided to call in.

'Have the results of my blood tests come in yet?' I

enquired at the reception desk.

'Yes, they're here,' replied the receptionist, checking through my case notes. She looked up, concerned. 'Are you all right, dear?' she asked. 'You don't look at all well.'

I explained about my weakness and loss of control.

'Well, surgery's finished, but Dr Billington's still here,' she said. 'I'll ask if he can see you.'

'Come in,' called the doctor a moment later as I knocked at his office door. 'Now, what's been happening to you?'

Once again I explained about the strange events of the morning. 'It's making normal life impossible,' I told him.

'Well, nothing's shown up in your blood tests,' he said. 'I wondered if the glandular fever you once had was flaring up again—the symptoms do recur sometimes, you know—but there's no sign of it.'

Dr Billington put down the blood test result and sat back in his chair, folding his arms. 'You need a long rest,' he said decisively. 'I'm going to sign you off work for another month.'

'I can't take a month off work!' I protested, astonished that he should even suggest it. 'The rehabilitation unit's been closed all summer while I was away—we only reopened today. I can't cancel the patients' appointments now.'

He gazed at me impassively from behind his cluttered desk.

'No, I can't take a month off,' I insisted. 'My keep-fit classes start this week. It's impossible!'

'Unless you take a month off work,' said the doctor, eyeing me firmly, 'you're going to be seriously ill.'

I took a month off work. By now it was becoming clear to me that something was very wrong.

'What does he say is the matter with you, then?' asked Peter who, used to an active, lively wife, was becoming increasingly irritated by my lying around the house for weeks on end.

'I don't know,' I snapped back, equally testily.

We were all feeling fed up with the situation. It was exhausting for me even to try to sit up straight. My head was constantly falling forwards on to my chest. What's more, the consultant was on his way to see me because my skin had turned yellow.

'I suspect there's something wrong with your blood,' the consultant said thoughtfully after examining me. 'It's time we got to the bottom of all this. I'd like you to come into hospital for tests.'

Two gruelling weeks later he came to see me with the results. 'We've given you a pretty thorough going over, Mrs Youngman,' he said, smiling encouragingly at me, 'and I'm pleased to say we can almost certainly rule out anything like cancer.'

Well, that was good news. The tests had ruled out a great many other things, too—but they hadn't actually discovered anything. I left with an appointment to see the liver specialist at one hospital and the psychiatrist at another. Perhaps one of *them* would be able to find out what was wrong with me.

'I need a change,' I said to Peter. 'I'm tired of doctors and illness. I think I'll go to the National Women's Register meeting tonight.'

'Good idea,' he said. 'You need something to cheer you up.'

I went, and found myself listening for most of the evening to Daphne, a new member, describing in graphic detail the symptoms of her illness. She sat wedged on the sofa between three other women, a diminutive figure in long black boots and wearing an enormous mohair sweater. She gave a dramatic account of the progressively debilitating disease she suffered from. It sounded rather like multiple sclerosis.

'The name of my illness,' she announced proudly, 'is myalgic encephalomyelitis!'

We were appalled! Whatever was wrong with me, I thought, couldn't possibly be as bad as that!

3

Mind over matter?

'Who are you?' I asked, puzzled at the sight of a strange face.

'I happen to be in charge of this ward,' came the frosty reply from the hospital sister. Then the frost melted into an encouraging smile. 'It's good to see you sitting up and taking notice again,' she said. 'You've been in a world of your own for over two days now.'

Two days! Could I possibly have deteriorated so much that I could lie for two days unaware of what was going on around me?

What had happened to change me from a cheerful, intelligent woman, determined to get well again so that I could pick up the threads of my disrupted life, into a panic-stricken creature, terrorised by horrific nightmares, lost for periods of time in a grey blankness of numb depression?

I suppose the first time I noticed any change in my usually positive attitude was while I was waiting to be admitted to the Intestinal Unit for tests on my liver.

Sheila, a friend, visited me, bringing with her a hypnosis tape designed to help people suffering from depression.

'But I don't feel depressed,' I insisted. 'It's my body that's sick, not my mind.'

'The doctors haven't found a physical cause for your illness yet,' she pointed out helpfully. 'Maybe you're depressed and don't recognise it.'

She had a point. After all, I'd been referred to a psychiatrist. I went to see him every week as an outpatient. Dr Johnstone was a delightful man, gentle and kind. So far, he had confined his treatment of me to half-hourly chats, not considering it necessary to use drugs or any other therapy.

'Well, I'm not going to let this thing beat me,' I declared. 'I don't care what's causing it—I just want to get back to normal life again.'

I meant it. I was desperate to be well again. If hypnosis could help I was willing to try it. In fact, I was willing to try anything!

My friend Susan came regularly to massage the palms of my hands and the soles of my feet using a technique called reflexology. I even bought a pair of special reflexology sandals which continued the treatment as you stood and walked. The inside sole was made up of tightly-clustered rubber prongs which thrust strongly into every part of your foot.

The sandals were agony to wear at first but I was determined to give anything, no matter how bizarre, a chance to work. So I persevered and, after the initial misery, got quite used to wearing them.

I bought myself a book on 'mind over matter'. If the doctors couldn't cure me, I thought, I would cure myself!

All through the Christmas holidays I lay on the studio sofa reading my book, learning how to meditate and practising psychic communication with some degree of success. The possibility of any of these strange spiritual practices being questionable or dangerous never crossed my mind.

'Try the tape, Chris,' persuaded Sheila. 'I really do find it most relaxing.'

'I'll try anything once,' I grinned, and as soon as she left I sat down to listen to it.

The hypnotist had a pleasant voice, soothing, peaceful, droning away in a relaxing monologue. I walked around the room enjoying the tranquillity but otherwise quite unaffected by him.

Then, all of a sudden, my mind was in uproar! Gone was the pleasant soothing effect. I was sobbing wildly in blind, unreasoning terror. I didn't know what was happening to me but, panic-stricken, I found myself phoning the doctor, crying, begging for help like a drowning person calling for a lifeline.

At that moment my mother arrived unexpectedly. For a split second she stood in the doorway, staring in astonishment, then, dumping her shopping bags on the floor, she turned and ran down the road to the doctor's surgery, bringing Dr Billington back with her. He stayed for half an hour, talking gently until I was calm again.

Perhaps that was when the change in my mental state began, but it was an isolated incident. By the time I was admitted to the Intestinal Unit in the new year I was my old self again, ready to chat and joke with the other patients, fully prepared to co-operate with the staff even though I knew the tests I would have to undergo were difficult and distressing.

I was in a ward with eighteen other patients, all extremely sick, some of them dying. The arrival of a physiotherapist as a fellow-patient caused quite a stir. As a medical person, I was expected to listen to detailed descriptions of their various symptoms and the treatments they had undergone in search of a cure. Each one vied with the other to give the most hair-raising account of the ordeal she had just experienced.

'O-o-h, that was awful,' Pauline would say, collapsing weakly on to the bed. 'The doctor was so rough! It's your turn soon, dear, isn't it? I hope you don't suffer as much as I did this afternoon.'

'It can't be as bad as that liver biopsy I had yesterday,' May would chip in. 'It was agony!'

The dreaded liver biopsy seemed to me the most fearful ordeal I would have to face. Larger-than-life descriptions flowed as freely as horrific tales of labour do in an antenatal clinic. The supposed terrors of the biopsy were blown up out of all proportion, yet they caused me to live in an agony of apprehension for days.

Fear seemed to have taken over my mind completely. Jumpy and nervous, I could no longer accept the tests stoically as a necessary ordeal but cried hysterically when the staff approached with yet another enormous needle and syringe to take a sample of blood.

One doctor seemed to be as nervous as I was. I watched as he fixed the needle on to the syringe, my stomach churning as he swabbed my bruised and punctured arm. As the needle drew near I flinched, screaming in pain as the startled doctor missed my vein and plunged the needle into the nerve.

'I'll be paralysed,' I sobbed, rubbing my throbbing arm. 'I'll never play the piano again!'

Later, I lay exhausted on the bed, miserable with fear about the terrible liver biopsy I was scheduled to endure that afternoon. All day long I waited, but no-one came to do the test. That evening Peter phoned the ward to ask how I was after undergoing the test, and the nurse informed him casually that it had been cancelled. No-one had remembered to tell me!

After two weeks on the unit I was discharged. Standing majestically at the foot of the bed, the specialist informed me from behind his big, black beard that he could find nothing wrong with my liver and he was transferring me to the blood specialist at the Royal Liverpool Hospital.

Unlike his registrar, who was convinced my problems were psychosomatic, the specialist did believe I was physically, not mentally, ill. He was an eminent man, skilled and very dedicated. Yet once again we had eliminated a great deal but found nothing. It was with much relief that I left one hospital and went straight into another.

The Royal Liverpool Hospital is a huge, multistorey building. I knew it well. I had applied for a job there—running a Rehabilitation Unit—just before we'd gone to France on holiday. When we got back the superintendent had rung to offer me the job, but I'd been reluctantly forced to turn it down. Before going away I had welcomed the challenge of extra responsibility. Now, I knew I could no longer manage even the running of our own home.

The blood specialist, Dr Richards, was a quiet, gentle man. In contrast to the high-pressure atmosphere of the Intestinal Unit where desperately ill people were treated with desperate measures, here life was taken at a more manageable pace.

The doctor took samples of my blood, mixed it with radioactive chromium and reintroduced it into my bloodstream. After the initial treatment I was able to go home. Elsa, a Finnish friend from a Women's Register group, drove me to the hospital every other day for scanning under a machine.

'I never thought I'd be radioactive!' I used to say jokingly. But by now I had very little left to joke about. Day by day I was growing weaker. I had been through so much, endured so many tests and investigations, and doctors were still no nearer finding out what was wrong with me.

Despite my weekly visits to Dr Johnstone at the Psychiatric Unit, fear was taking hold of every part of my life.

I was now more afraid of living than of dying, so I made up my mind. I couldn't bear to live this way any longer. On my next visit to the hospital I would climb to the very top of that enormous multistorey building and throw myself off.

4

The last straw

'Mum, are you all right?'

Sally was standing in the bedroom doorway, fiddling nervously with the strap of her schoolbag. I burrowed my face into the pillow and ignored her. It was already after nine o'clock, but still she hovered uncertainly, not wanting to leave until she was sure I could cope alone.

'Can I get you anything?' she asked, 'A cup of tea or something?'

'Oh, leave me alone!' I shouted irritably. 'Go to school.'

Her face fell but still she didn't leave. Poor Sally. She was only fourteen but she often bore the brunt of my wild emotional swings. As my illness progressed we were gradually to exchange roles, she caring for me as a mother would care for a fractious, sick child.

The dilemma she faced this morning was typical of the sort of thing she often had to cope with.

She stood half in, half out of the doorway, acutely aware of the time but reluctant to go while I still lay sobbing in bed. Then the doorbell rang, sending a relieved Sally winging down the stairs. She hoped it would be a friend calling who would keep me company so that she could go to school with a clear conscience. It was, in fact, a neighbour, Liz, who stood on the doorstep. She was obviously in a state of great agitation.

'Is your mum in?' she asked urgently.

'Well, yes,' said Sally, no longer sure this was the rescuer she had hoped for. 'She's not feeling too good but I'll tell her you're here.'

She dashed back up the stairs to my room. 'Liz is here, Mum,' she said. 'She seems a bit upset.'

My heart sank. I felt depressed enough already without listening to someone else's problems. Only that morning I'd rung the doctor's surgery asking routine questions about the dosage of my tablets but really longing to blurt out how desperate I felt. Instead I'd just replaced the receiver and cried as if my heart would break.

But a medical training dies hard. I was used to listening to other people's problems—it was an everyday part of my job. So I put on my dressing-gown and slippers and staggered downstairs to see what was wrong.

'Chris, something awful's happened,' cried Liz, rushing to meet me as I came into the hall. 'Do you remember Doris who was in the general ward with you before Christmas?'

I thought hard for a moment. I'd been in so many hospital wards by now that it was difficult to remember everybody. 'Do you mean the wife of your driving instructor?' I asked curiously, wondering what on earth could have happened to make Liz so upset.

'That's right,' she said. 'She had to have her leg amputated. She's been absolutely devastated about it.'

I nodded understandingly. I knew from my work in the Rehabilitation Unit how traumatic the loss of a limb could be.

'But not only that,' Liz went on. 'Her husband was depressed and he couldn't cope with the news. He committed suicide today.'

Tears brimmed in her eyes as she struggled to keep her self-control; she looked stunned by the shock.

'Oh, Chris,' she said miserably. 'He hung himself!'

I felt sick. Suicide! For days now my mind had been filled with thoughts of how I could kill myself. Drugs, razor-blades, exhaust fumes—all sorts of possibilities had chased each other around my mind.

But I wanted something certain. Something from which there could be no reprieve—I wanted no well-meaning interference at the last moment. In my mind's eye I pictured the tall hospital building where I would secretly make my jump. Yes, I knew what I was going to do. But here was someone who had actually done it.

I put my arm around Liz's shoulder, sympathetically. 'Let me make you some coffee,' I said, leading her into the kitchen. I needed a cup myself. Already emotionally battered, I found Liz's distress too much for me to handle. I felt as if I could take no more.

As we walked through the door a jet plane roared overhead, rattling the house to its very foundations. The noise was ear-splitting. I crashed on to the red quarry-tiled floor, shaking, quite unable to get up. I lay there, my heart pounding wildly, terrified by the shock.

As the sound faded into the distance, Liz and Sally gently helped me to my feet and we walked shakily into the dining-room where I curled up in the big old armchair by the fire.

'I think *I'd* better make that cup of coffee,' said Liz
weakly. Sally, white-faced and scared, followed her into
the kitchen.

I was scared too. Fear—constant fear—seemed to fill my
mind, yet I couldn't explain why. I didn't know what
I was afraid of! I felt strange sitting there, curiously
detached from what was going on around me.

In the distance I heard the doorbell ringing, voices
murmuring in the hall—then Dr Billington was beside
me, talking gently. I gazed at him wonderingly, puzzled
at how he could have got here so soon.

'No,' he explained, 'no-one sent for me. I thought there
was something wrong when I spoke to you on the
telephone this morning. I just called to see you.'

What a good doctor he was. Even though I couldn't
explain how I was feeling, he'd read between the lines
of our conversation and taken the time to visit me. His
thoughtfulness had brought him to me just when I needed
him most.

I know the trend is to complain about the National
Health Service with its waiting lists and cuts and
supposedly indifferent general practitioners, but that was
never my experience. Despite the fact that I was ill for
a long time with a rare disease which never responded
for more than a few weeks to any treatment, no-one ever
gave up on me. I always received the very best of care.

Liz brought in the coffee then went back to the kitchen
to turn her attention to Sally. Faced with someone in
greater need than herself, Liz had become a tower of

strength.

'Are you all right, Sally?' she asked kindly, her heart going out to the dejected girl. 'I expect things are a bit difficult for you at the moment.'

Sally nodded, taken by surprise. People didn't usually ask how *she* was—Mum was the one they worried about.

'You're very late for school,' Liz observed, looking at the clock. 'How are you getting on these days? Are you managing to do your homework?'

'Oh, school's all right, but the homework is difficult to get through,' admitted Sally. 'By the time we've done the housework or visited Mum if she's in hospital, there's not much time left for homework. Mum's too ill and Dad's too busy to help me, but I usually manage to get through it in the end.'

'Do the teachers know how ill your mum is?' persisted Liz.

'I tried to tell them,' answered Sally, 'but they didn't seem interested.'

'Well, I'm interested,' declared Liz firmly. 'If ever you need any help, just remember I'm always there.'

While Liz was comforting Sally, Dr Billington was talking to me. It was such a relief to be able to unburden myself. I poured out all my fears.

'I'm so frightened, doctor,' I confessed. 'All I can think about is killing myself! I keep going over all the different ways of doing it.'

No sign of shock or surprise showed on his face. He spoke in a very matter-of-fact way, as if he were asking about my plans for the holidays.

'Have you decided on a particular way?' he asked.

'Oh, yes,' I replied calmly. 'The next time I go to the Royal Liverpool Hospital for scanning I'm going to climb the fire escape to the top of the building and jump. No-one will see me round at the back of the hospital—I don't want some do-gooder trying to stop me.'

He sat back in his chair, observing me thoughtfully.

'Could I use your phone, please?' he asked suddenly, and left the room. He came back a few minutes later and sat down again.

'I've just been speaking to Dr Johnstone at the Psychiatric Unit,' he said quietly. 'At the moment we feel that the emotional side of your illness—the depression—is in far more urgent need of help than the physical aspects.'

He paused. The room was completely still, the silence broken only by the squabbling of birds outside the window. I waited trustingly for him to speak. No matter what it might cost I wanted to get better, though I could guess what he was going to suggest.

He shuffled his feet awkwardly on the carpet. 'Dr Johnstone and I agree that the best possible thing for you is to admit you to the Psychiatric Unit as an in-patient.'

I put my head down on the chair arm and cried with relief. At last someone was going to help me!

Then I realised: I'd finally had a nervous breakdown.

5

Inside the window

'This isn't real. It can't be happening to me,' I thought, scarcely able to believe that I was now an in-patient at a Psychiatric Unit. I didn't belong here. I was physically, not mentally ill!

I looked around fearfully at my fellow-patients, a desperate group of schizophrenics and manic-depressives, and wondered how I could possibly manage to stay sane if I were in such company for any length of time.

Some, I supposed, like the emaciated anorexics, were short-term patients like myself. Others, drooling old men and women suffering the ravages of senile dementia, had become so violent and unpredictable that they would probably never go home again.

'I'm not mad,' I told myself fiercely, over and over again. 'This is all a bad dream. If I can just hang on, I'll soon be out of here.'

I curled up in an armchair that first day, dazed and homesick, my mind blanking out the reality of where I was.

After evening visiting I made my first friend, James, a man whose illness took the form of sudden, violent behaviour against himself. Only weeks before, he'd had to undergo emergency surgery after stabbing himself

several times in the stomach. Looking at him now, with
his hand stretched out in welcome as he introduced
himself, I could scarcely believe him capable of such an act.

'What job did you do before you were ill?' he asked
as we chatted together.

I blushed in embarrassment. 'I—er—actually was a senior
physiotherapist,' I admitted, waiting for his shocked
reaction.

'We have a lot in common,' he replied ruefully. 'I was
a doctor.'

Our days in the Psychiatric Unit were mapped out for
us as rigidly as a school timetable. Apart from our
consultations with the doctors, we had group activities
several times a week. Art therapy and keep-fit were
compulsory. No matter how weak or ill I might be feeling,
some member of staff would bustle along and rout me
out of the bed or chair I was resting in.

'Come along, Chris!' they'd say cheerfully, handing me
a box of tissues to mop up my never-ending stream of
tears. 'Keep-fit is good for you. It helps bounce you out
of your depression.'

One of the strangest physical manifestations of my
illness was the way I could collapse without warning.
Walking along a corridor, or in the middle of a keep-fit
session or therapy group, all strength would suddenly
leave me. My legs would buckle and I'd sink to the ground
if there was nowhere to sit down quickly.

Any physical exertion, such as the keep-fit sessions,
could bring on such an attack and, although the trained
staff were sympathetic, some of the student or auxiliary

nurses would sweep scornfully by as I lay on the floor. It hurt to think that they assumed I was seeking attention, but as the attacks struck without warning there was nothing I could do about it.

Art therapy sessions were always traumatic. It was here that we were expected to reveal our innermost feelings through the medium of paper and paint.

Catherine, the occupational therapist who led the group, was a tall, fair woman who devoted hours of her own time to helping us understand what we were trying to express through our artistic efforts. First we would paint something which represented the way we felt at the moment. Then, after discussing our feelings together, we would go back and paint how we would like our lives to be.

'Draw your fears,' we were instructed.

It was like lighting a short fuse. I immediately produced a horrific painting of faces yelling at me from a sky thick with storm-clouds. Huge jackboots trampled me underfoot as I lay drowning in the sea.*

Being forced to think about my fears was such a nightmare that, like most of the other patients, I ended up in tears. I longed to escape, to shut out the awful reality of what we had been discussing. But escape was impossible as the doors were always locked during these sessions.

Only once was I so terrified that I actually managed to unlock the door and burst out of the room. I stood

---

* This painting is reproduced on the back cover.

outside in the corridor, leaning against the cool walls until I felt able to go back in and face the rest of the session.

I'd been in the unit about a month when a letter arrived for me.

'Look at this, Peter,' I exclaimed, producing a printed leaflet. 'It's from Daphne. Do you remember me meeting her at the Women's Register evening?'

'The woman with the unpronounceable illness?'

'Yes. Myalgic encephalomyelitis.' I handed over the leaflet.

He read it thoughtfully.

'Chris, the symptoms described in this leaflet are exactly the same as yours,' he said with alarm. 'It's a rare disease but I think we should show this to the doctor.'

I showed it first to James and asked his opinion. 'It sounds as though this could be it,' he agreed soberly. 'I would definitely let Dr Peacock see it.'

I handed over the leaflet to Dr Peacock, the registrar, at our next consultation and watched in dismay as he pushed it into my file, having barely glanced at it. He was one of the growing band of medical staff who believed there was nothing physically wrong with me and who concentrated all their efforts on curing my depression.

I never saw the leaflet again.

Days turned into weeks. Patients came and went, helped by their short stay in the unit and able to return to normal family life. But I remained.

I felt trapped. Inwardly I was the same person, but instead of living life I had become an observer, looking out at others through a glass wall which I was powerless to break through.

My days were filled with unimaginable horror, panic and helpless sobbing. My nights were terrorised by violent nightmares. My only consolation was in playing the battered old piano. Hidden away in a small room at the end of the corridor, I played most evenings, clinging to my one surviving link with sanity.

Then came Mother's Day. We in the unit knew that all over the country families would be celebrating together with flowers and cards and special treats. We were no exception. All those who were able went home for the day, and Peter arrived to pick me up.

James came, too—we had arranged to take him to visit his family. We drove to his big old house and were invited to have coffee with his lovely wife and their tiny baby. Soon their other children arrived back from church bearing little bunches of flowers.

They sat together on the sofa, outwardly a perfectly normal family but in reality living under the sinister shadow of an illness which could strike at any moment, destroying any chance of happiness. On the way out we passed through the big square hallway with its great mahogany banister. This had been the scene of James' dramatic bid for freedom when, at Christmas, he'd been taken ill. Pursued by police and ambulance-men, he'd rushed madly up the stairs. Finding himself cornered, he had launched himself from the top of the banister, slid down the huge Christmas tree and landed flat on his back amid the shattered baubles!

Promising to call later to pick James up and take him back to hospital with us, we drove on to my mother's house.

She and my aunt made us poached eggs and we had two slices of her special Mother's Day cake. Suddenly, in the midst of all the chatter and fun, I felt the dreaded icy numbness spreading through me and I collapsed.

'Take me back to the hospital,' I pleaded, though I knew we were supposed to be out for the whole day. 'I want to go back!'

'I can't take you back yet, love,' said Peter. 'You'll be all right in a few minutes.'

'Well, take me home then,' I insisted desperately.

So, leaving behind a distressed and bewildered mother and aunt, we went home. The swiftness with which the illness could overcome me was infuriating. One minute I would be all right, the next lying on the floor, weak and helpless.

Feeling very ill, I sat stroking our guinea-pig, the day's celebrations forgotten, wanting only to go back to the hospital. Peter, who had cleaned the house from top to bottom in preparation for my homecoming and had made a special dinner with a real pineapple as the centrepiece, sat and wept with despair.

'I *will* get better, Peter,' I said, trying to reassure him. 'Everyone else is able to go home after a few weeks—I'm sure I'll be well enough soon.'

But he shook his head, no longer able to play such games of make-believe. Sally came home from the riding stables, mucky and smelly from the horses, but I grabbed her and hugged her anyway and we cried together as she gave me some flowers and a beautiful Mother's Day card she'd made.

Peter prepared the dinner and we all enjoyed it, especially the pineapple. I was feeling a little better by the time we collected James and drove back to the hospital, laden with flowers and bags of clean washing.

No-one knew of the great wave of relief that swept over me as I re-entered the ward. It had become part of my life. I had a beautiful home, a family who loved me, numerous concerned friends and colleagues and a fulfilling career waiting for me—but I was only secure enough to cope with life within the confines of a mental hospital.

6

Trapped!

He was gaining on me. I knew it without even looking back to see how close he was. Running madly through the labyrinth of corridors, I felt his evil presence growing stronger as the distance between us narrowed.

For one heart-stopping moment I thought the corridor was a dead-end—then I spotted the spiral staircase, twisting its way ornately to the very top of the building. I kept on running, up and up, round and round, heart pounding, lungs bursting as my breath came in great, painful gasps.

I was at the top of the staircase, whirling round, searching desperately for a way out, only to realise that I was trapped.

He walked slowly towards me, smiling cruelly as he forced me back against the curving metal bars of the gigantic circular birdcage, twisting, pulling at the fringing on the Indian silk scarf around my neck.

I shook the metal bars of my cage, screaming in terror as the devil reached out and jerked me towards him.

I woke to find my nightdress soaked in sweat, the sheets twisted and screwed up, the blankets falling off the bed. But despite the relief of knowing it was just a nightmare, the terror was still with me, vivid and real.

I got out of bed and paced up and down the corridor,

trying to calm my jangling nerves before facing the long
hours of lying awake, waiting for the Psychiatric Unit
to crash into life again. It was no use. I was too afraid
to go back to bed. I made my way to the nurses' station
and joined the little night-nurse at her desk until the fear
receded enough for me to face going back to the darkened
ward.

These violent nightmares were hard to handle—reality
was nightmare enough without having imaginary fears
and traumas to cope with while snatching what little drug-
induced sleep I could get.

'Chris, do you know old Rodney's asleep in your bed?'
asked Wendy, one of the patients, as we queued up for
our nightly handout of sleeping-pills. Abandoning my
place in the queue, I went into the dormitory and my
heart sank when I saw the filthy mess this demented old
geriatric had made of my sheets and nightdress.

The nurses quickly removed him and stripped and
remade the bed while I washed my nightdress. We
patients were surprisingly tolerant of each other's eccentric
behaviour, knowing that we in turn would need tolerance
with our own unusual or difficult ways.

By a strange coincidence, as I sat in the television lounge
that evening watching *News at Ten* and waiting for my
nightdress to dry, the newsreader reported that the Queen
had had a similar experience: an intruder had broken into
her bedroom in Buckingham Palace.

'You're in good company, Chris!' grinned the other
patients.

'That's right,' I said. 'She'd probably be safer in here

with us!'

Another source of petty irritation was the kleptomaniac in our midst. It was obvious there was one, but none of us knew which patient was the culprit.

'Chris, that sweater you knitted for me has been stolen!' cried Ada, in great distress.

'Are you sure?' I asked, helping her to check her locker. But it had definitely gone and we never saw it again. It was uncanny how stealthily the thief managed to spirit away our few precious belongings without ever being seen by either patients or staff.

One afternoon, as I lay on my bed resting after a tiring trip into Chester, I fell asleep. When I woke up, the book Peter had been reading to me during visiting time had mysteriously vanished from my locker.

'I'm fed up with this!' I declared, getting really agitated. 'That's a bar of chocolate, half a box of tissues, a bottle of perfume, my new white blouse, a sweater and now even my book!'

No possession was too worthless to be of interest to our kleptomaniac, so I took to carrying all my belongings around with me in a cloth bag, the only exception being my raincoat, which was too big. The ward sister took pity on me and put it in her locker, which, unlike ours, actually did lock. I went around hoping she would be on duty when it rained!

Looking back at the time I spent in the unit, I'm always amazed at the patience, love and sense of humour the nurses showed towards us. Bizzare incidents were everyday occurrences. Violence and hysterics were commonplace. Quieter periods were always treated with suspicion, for they usually proved to be the proverbial calm before the storm.

One peaceful afternoon I returned from my therapy group to find the lounge in absolute chaos. It was like a pantomime in there! One old man was strutting about with a vase of flowers; another had gone completely beserk and was creating havoc, first in his room, then in someone else's bed.

Meanwhile, some of the other patients were so confused they didn't know which were bedrooms and which were toilets and had been urinating on the floor. One old lady sat like a rock, refusing to be moved and fighting wildly if anyone tried to touch her.

The perspiring staff were wrestling in the stiflingly hot and humid air to get their new intake of patients under control.

'Where have they all come from?' I asked in bewilderment.

'Some of the nurses at another hospital are on strike,' explained Roger, the male nurse, as he leaned breathlessly against the doorpost for a moment. 'We've had to take in these extra patients to help the remaining staff cope.'

That afternoon, the nurses dealt with their unruly charges with a professionalism and kindness which impressed me, ill as I was, rousing me to indignation that caring people such as these should be forced into taking strike action to earn a reasonable wage.

Fortunately, not every day was as chaotic as that one. On Thursday nights some sort of entertainment was usually organised for us.

Disco night caused a few folk to feel a bit apprehensive, especially the old ladies among us. 'I can't go to a *disco,'* one grumbled to another. 'I'm too old for all this new-fangled dancing.' But after much hesitation the entire ward agreed to go and we ambled along there together.

The atmosphere was depressingly flat at first as patients lined the walls, weeping and withdrawn, for we had long since forgotten how to enjoy ourselves properly. But as the evening went on we began to relax and have a good time. Our medication released us from our inhibitions.

The evening ended with the young men dancing a cancan in the middle of the floor, the rest of us gathered around them in a circle, clapping and shouting, 'Come on, lads, come on!'

The funniest social event I attended, however, was the ceilidh. A wonderful group of men arrived with an organ, a violin, an accordion and drums. At the beginning of the evening they tried to organise the patients to dance a simple progressive barn dance in groups of eight.

Never in all my years of attending square dances have I seen anything like the muddle they managed to create. At one stage everyone was swinging with everyone else in a single, gigantic tangle. The groups were unknotted and reformed into eights and the dance restarted. But it quickly became more and more mangled as the music progressed until, after about sixteen bars, the dance ground to a halt.

The fellow in charge kept shouting, 'Now where did you all go wrong?' as if he couldn't believe it was possible to mess up such a simple dance.

Wisely, he abandoned any further attempt at keeping order, simply announced the name of each dance and played the music through to the end despite the fact that most patients, exhausted by their first efforts, were slumped against the walls ignoring him.

Then, suddenly, all in the room were on their feet, ready to join in again. The group leader had announced the *Gay Gordons,* and this was the one and only dance we all felt we could have a reasonable shot at. I found myself dancing with a lively pensioner called Dora who, despite having Parkinson's Disease, danced her way round the room in bare feet with a thick bandage wound around her big toe!

I usually enjoyed the social evenings and joined in unless I was particularly withdrawn or unwell. But always, as I watched the other patients, I was conscious of not really being mentally ill in the way they were. I was certain that the signs of mental illness which I showed were a direct result of a physical ailment, and the longing to be well enough to go home again was an almost intolerable burden of grief inside me.

When the weekends came, however, and Peter wanted to take me home for a visit, fear would overcome me. It would build up bit by bit as the day went on until he arrived to collect me, when he would find that after a hard day's work he now had to cope with my distress at having to leave the ward and go home with him.

'Would you like to go home with your husband for the weekend?' enquired one young nurse innocently, causing me to erupt in a volcanic display of aggression.

'No!' I screamed. 'Leave me alone, leave me alone!'

Red-hot rage surged up inside me as I hurled myself at the wardrobes and lockers in the dormitory, furiously trying to smash them to pieces. On this particular day I'd been out to the swimming-pool and come back tired to find I'd missed both my tea and the drugs round. So my reactions were even more over-the-top than usual.

I tore my clothes from their hangers and piled them into my case, then threw myself on top of it screaming hysterically.

'I feel so ill! Why can't I get better? I'm a failure! I just want to die!'

All at once my legs gave way and I landed on the floor with a bump.

Now I wanted to scream with frustration. Struggling to my feet, I slammed the ward door nearly off its hinges, stormed my way through the lounge full of staring patients and out to the waiting car. I collapsed into the front seat and huddled down, totally switching myself off from Peter, who wearily got in beside me and drove home.

Sally was waiting eagerly for us and came running to the door to welcome me home. My heart went out to her, but the creature I had become swept by, ignoring her, wanting only to hide in the depths of my bed.

Brim full of hate and intensely lonely, I cried into my pillow, 'Help me, God, help me! Nobody else can.' But there was no reply, no word of comfort from heaven as I lay exhausted and sobbed myself to sleep.

I awoke at five o'clock the next morning trembling from head to foot, and realised I hadn't taken any drugs since lunchtime the previous day. I knew the withdrawal symptoms would be pretty bad because sometimes I'd secretly tried to reduce my dosage in an attempt to wean myself off them.

The ward sister had once spotted me trembling and dropping things, and warned me sharply never to try to stop taking the drugs without medical supervision.

By the time Peter had got me back to the hospital for the nine o'clock drug handout the trembling had turned to violent shaking. So I went along to the relaxation class and lay on the bed there, my body jerking uncontrollably, my organs seeming to shake inside me, until—almost three hours later—the drugs took effect and the withdrawal symptoms faded away.

'What's happened to me?' I wondered miserably. 'Who am I?'

When I looked into the mirror the reflection was more or less mine. Haggard maybe, thin and tired, but still recognisably me. But when I looked inside myself, the person I used to be had gone. The real Chris Youngman had died and a stranger had taken my place.

I stumbled into the lounge and found the entire ward riveted to the television set, quiet for once as they sat in total concentration. I sat down among them, curious to see what they were watching.

The scene on the TV screen was strangely familiar. The programme was a documentary about life in a Psychiatric Unit! I felt sickened, utterly revolted. The mentally ill watching in fascination a programme about mental illness.

I wanted to kick the screen in.

7

A ray of hope

Spring had turned reluctantly into summer when the first glimmer of hope began to dawn in our lives.

Overcome with a new desire to go home, I set about persuading Peter to decorate the house before I was discharged. I had no reason to suppose this would be soon, as my depression continued. I still needed high doses of antidepressant drugs to see me through each day, but I was due for a routine consultation with Dr Johnstone and I was ever hopeful of a new treatment or drug which would release me from the prison in which I'd become trapped.

'Dr Johnstone wants to see you, too, this week, Peter,' I told him one evening during the visiting hour. 'I've been here for six months now.'

He needed no reminding of that. The strain showed in the taut lines on his face. Usually he sat beside my bed in the evenings, so weary that he was barely able to speak, but tonight he seemed excited.

'I heard something today, Chris,' he said eagerly. 'I was up the ladder, painting the ceiling in the front room, listening to *Woman's Hour* on the radio. A doctor was speaking about food allergies. The case being discussed,' he went on, 'was a woman whose symptoms were similar to yours. She was cured when her doctor put her on a dairy-product-free diet!'

It was the first new angle we'd had for weeks. We discussed the possibility of my being well again soon, and Peter went home that evening with a lighter heart than he'd had for a long time. He planned to ask Dr Johnstone about the diet when he saw him later in the week. But when actually faced with Dr Johnstone in the consulting room, Peter found that before he could explain what was on his mind the interview was at an end.

He decided instead to speak to our family doctor, Dr Billington, a man with whom he had already built a good relationship and who, he felt sure, would listen to his suggestion with an open mind.

'She's not *still* in there, is she?' gasped the doctor in amazement when Peter approached him. He listened as Peter explained his frustration at my lack of progress and put forward the idea of trying me on a dairy-product-free diet.

'Well, you could try it,' he said doubtfully, 'but you'd find it almost impossible to put into practice. Milk is used in all kinds of foods—things you'd never imagine. Even sausages!'

But we were determined at least to give the diet a try. It worked for some people, so why not for me? Our main difficulty would be in controlling what I ate while I was still in hospital. Many of the staff there, firmly convinced that my illness was simply an offshoot of my depression, were unlikely to put the kitchen staff to a lot of trouble and extra work in making up a complicated diet.

The problem was solved, however, in a most unexpected way. The nurses decided to go on strike!

All patients—except the few really dangerous ones— were to be sent home into the care of their relatives. It meant that we were on our own. Peter could supervise what I ate and we could try the new diet.

As Dr Billington had predicted, we had a lot of trouble finding the right kind of foods, especially a milk substitute. But we persevered and discovered to our delight that by the end of the week I felt much better. In fact, I was well enough to drive myself to the hospital!

I arrived for my routine consultation with Dr Johnstone just in time to see the nurses staggering out with their banners to picket the gates. Inside was chaos. The picketing had obviously been effective. Hardly any food was getting through to the kitchens, so the patients who had remained behind were having a rough time.

Dr Johnstone was rushing about frantically looking for his big black diary which had been lost in the confusion and without which he was quite unable to organise his busy schedule.

He was impressed when he saw me. I was wearing my smartest Harrods' blouse. I obviously looked and felt much better.

'I'm pleased with you,' he said, when we'd had time to talk together. 'You're far better than I expected you to be.' He looked genuinely delighted—he'd never had occasion to praise me before! I raced with tears of joy in my eyes to Sister's office to tell her the news.

'He's sending me to an allergy specialist,' I told the staff excitedly, 'Dr King at the Royal Liverpool.' I drove home feeling more hopeful than I had for a long time.

Still on cloud nine, I wanted to do something practical to help my fellow-patients left back at the hospital. I went into the kitchen and, looking through the freezer, discovered lots of apples left over from the autumn. I set to work and soon had a great cauldron of stewed apples spitting and boiling on the stove. I worked non-stop for three hours and by four o'clock had made enough pies to feed all seventy-two patients and staff on the ward.

We loaded the pies on to the back seat of the car. Not wanting my hard work to be confiscated by the pickets, I covered them with a blanket and sneaked them through the back door into the ward.

Exhausted, but thrilled at what I had achieved, I drove home convinced that we really were on to something. The new diet had accomplished more than I would ever have dared hope for. I lay on the sofa feeling pleased with myself while Peter tackled the battlefield in the kitchen.

Before long the phone rang. It was the ward sister, ringing to tell us that every delicious pie had been eaten and enjoyed by the patients and staff. I lay back, grinning smugly, while Peter wailed forlornly, 'The pies might have gone but the mess hasn't!'

I spent the whole of the next day recovering from my exertions, my throbbing legs propped on cushions as I lazed in the garden, reliving the moment on the ward earlier that day when one hungry young doctor, biting into a huge slice of pie, remarked, 'We'll have to cure you more often!'

But on Monday morning I felt ill again. I was back in the hospital ward lying on my bed, all the hope and strength of the previous week gone.

The staff, however, encouraged by my sudden progress, had decided to discharge me. The doctor sat on the end of my bed, insisting that I could now cope at home. But I felt frightened at the thought of being abandoned in my present state. My joints were weak and aching and my head hurt, as if my brain were covered in sores. I couldn't even concentrate long enough to read a book any more. So I stayed firmly put, refusing to leave the security of my bed.

'Chris, you must go home now,' insisted the doctor. 'Don't you see? You'll never be able to live a normal life again unless you can make a start outside the unit. Go home and don't come back except for your outpatient appointments.'

I was shaking all over, my dignity drowned in the terror which threatened to submerge me.

'You must learn to live again, Chris,' the doctor said firmly. 'Don't come back to the ward, even if you feel suicidal.'

I gathered up my belongings and made my way out of the door. The wind, gusting strongly, slammed it behind me. I walked across the wind-blown grass towards the hospital gates feeling I'd lost all hope of ever finding my identity again. Six months in a mental hospital—a whole year since I'd first become ill, yet we were apparently no nearer finding a solution. All we could do now was stick to my new diet and wait to see what Dr

King would have to say when he saw me.

Before that day arrived, another event came up: the Great Wirral Marathon. Peter was a regular runner and had signed up for the race. Fortunately, I felt well enough to go and cheer him along the route—twenty-six miles of it.

He was eager to be away, his number stitched to his singlet back and front, and the final touch—cooking oil—applied between his toes. A fearsome army gun was produced, ready to signal the start. Someone announced over the loudspeaker that if the gun failed to go off a whistle would blow instead, but everything went according to plan. There was a BANG! and they were off.

Cars and policemen were everywhere as we followed the route, stopping at strategic points to cheer the competitors on. Peter passed the thirteen-mile halfway point running well. We drove on to the finishing line and waited excitedly to see the first runners arriving.

Then at last Peter came into view, turning the final corner and staggering towards the finish. He looked in an absolutely desperate state.

On the opposite side of the road one of the crowd nudged her neighbour and pointed at him. 'Poor thing!' she exclaimed sympathetically. Despite all my problems, I couldn't resist a chuckle.

Peter lay on the grass by the finishing line, totally exhausted.

'Never again,' he gasped, just as he had done the year before!

Eventually the day arrived that I'd looked forward to

for so long—my appointment with the allergy specialist, Dr King. I was ushered into the consulting room. There behind the desk was the man on whom I was pinning all my hopes, flanked on either side by doctors, students and several nurses.

He began by asking me a question. Ill at ease with so many spectators present, I mumbled an answer.

'She's a bit slow, isn't she?' he remarked to the room in general.

'What?' I exclaimed angrily.

'I was just saying you are a bit slow,' he repeated carefully, as if to a dimwitted child.

'If you'd just spent six months in a Psychiatric Unit you probably wouldn't be so lively yourself!' I retorted hotly.

'Ah, she can be quite dynamic after all,' he declared, amused by my indignation.

In the light of our further discussion he decided to restrict me to a very limited diet for three months. If I improved enough, he would see me again and 'make me better'.

That was the last straw. I burst into tears.

'Four consultants have already promised to make me better,' I cried, 'but none of them have!'

He gazed at me, startled, as my panic spilled out.

'You were my last hope,' I sobbed. 'I wish I were dead!'

Dr King asked about my work as a physiotherapist and I told him I'd been offered a job as a senior physiotherapist running the Rehabilitation Unit in this very hospital. I'd been forced to refuse it because I was too ill to work any more.

I described my present life, where I was passed from one hospital to another within the group. I told him how I'd pinned all my hopes on Dr Johnstone, but still my nightmare went on.

There was silence in the room, the atmosphere charged with tension as we all waited for Dr King to speak.

'Many people have come to me as their last hope,' he said finally, 'and they are now well.'

I looked into his face and knew that I could trust him. Somehow, despite his initial attitude towards me, a bond had grown between us.

8

A change of direction

Christmas saw me back in hospital again. Three months had gone by since I'd last seen Dr King. They had been three long and difficult months of rigidly following the restricted diet he had given me, all the time wondering if this really was the key to my return to health. If not, we were trudging our way wearily down yet another blind alley.

'What shall we do if the allergy diagnosis is wrong?' I asked Dr Billington anxiously.

'I really don't know,' he replied honestly.

I almost despaired trying to follow that diet.

'I'm no cook!' I wailed, when faced with an impossible menu which allowed virtually none of the usual foods we ate.

A cookery book arrived in the post, sent by the hospital dietitian. I leafed through its pages then decided to try the gingerbread recipe. It didn't look too difficult.

I started to weigh out the ingredients. There seemed to be an awful lot of them just to make one cake. I got out a bigger bowl and transferred everything into that. On the stove bubbled a whole tin of treacle mixed with hot oil.

'What are you doing, Mum?' asked Sally, coming into

the kitchen holding in her arms Rosemary the guinea-pig and her five wriggling babies.

'Making a cake from this new diet recipe book,' I muttered distractedly. 'Pass me another bowl, Sally—this one isn't big enough either.'

I put the dry ingredients into the bigger bowl and rushed across to give the boiling treacle another stir.

'Will you keep an eye on these for me?' Sally casually dumped the five tiny babies into the now empty bowl. 'I'm cleaning their cage out.'

I weighed the rest of the ingredients. 'Surely this can't be right,' I exclaimed, as the bowl started to overflow again. I shifted it all into my breadmaking bowl, wondering if I had a cake tin big enough.

I poured the oil and treacle in. 'Beat well,' I read, peering at the sticky recipe book and pushing aside the jars of guinea-pig food which had somehow found their way over to my side of the kitchen.

'Oh, Sally, I can't manage with all these,' I groaned, as she reappeared with Emma, our other guinea-pig, and her three babies. 'Take some of them upstairs to Dad. He's gone to run a bath—he can look after them up there.'

When I looked back at my cake mix, something had happened to it. Like a scene from *Alice in Wonderland* it had shrunk to a tiny leaden ball, lost in the bottom of that enormous bowl. I pulled it out in gluey strands, laughing helplessly as I transferred the glutinous mess to my smallest cake tin. Sally, who hadn't heard me laugh for a long time, became quite hysterical.

'Oh, please let me take it to show the girls at school,'

she begged, when the solid, brick-like cake came out of the oven. It certainly wasn't fit to eat—we could hardly get it out of the tin.

She came home the next day with a plaster on her finger. 'I cut myself on your cake!' she announced indignantly.

The diet was certainly helping, but the hoped-for miracle wasn't taking place. By the time the three-month trial period was over and we went back to see Dr King, the allergy specialist, my reactions were so slow I could hardly speak properly.

'Ask her husband to come in,' he told the nurse, giving up on his attempts to communicate with me. I sat like a rag doll in the chair, listening as they discussed me, too weak to be able to speak for myself.

'Your wife is suffering from a rare disease called myalgic encephalomyelitis,' Dr King told Peter. 'We call it M.E. for short. I'd like to admit her to my ward tomorrow to investigate her allergies. They are being caused by her illness.'

So we'd been right all along! Our very worst fears were realised. We now knew for certain that I had an incurable disease, one so rare that most doctors barely acknowledged its existence.

I felt only peace as I heard the diagnosis. At least I wasn't mentally ill. I wasn't a hypochondriac. Everything I'd experienced was the result of a genuine illness, not the product of an over-active imagination. Despite the awesomeness of what we had just been told I could only feel relief.

On the way home we stopped at the Psychiatric Unit and told the ward sister what we had just learnt. She was obviously aghast, but quickly recovered her professional smile and offered a few helpful words of advice.

The sooty bricks of the hospital buildings looked grubby and uninviting when we arrived there the following morning in the December sleet. Ward A2 was hidden away somewhere in the centre. A small, plastic Christmas tree crouched in the hallway, a dismal reminder of the fun and festivities we should have been preparing for.

I'd hardly finished stuffing my locker with knitting-wool and the rest of my belongings when a small, ginger-haired doctor arrived to begin my tests.

She injected me with a tiny amount of milk and immediately I felt ill. After a while I couldn't walk. Soon after that I couldn't talk. Later in the day, when I'd recovered, I was given food—a chemical mixture with the consistency of slush, flavoured with a sickly sweet, pink powder. I was to live on this for a week.

'Thank goodness they've promised I'll be home for Christmas!' I thought, after tasting it.

In the new year, Beth, a social worker from the hospital, came to visit me to discuss the possibility of our having a downstairs toilet fitted. I was getting too weak to manage the exhausting journeys up and down the stairs to the bathroom.

'There should be no problem getting a grant to cover the cost of the work,' she said. 'Now you're getting invalidity benefit it should be paid for automatically.'

How I'd battled with my pride over applying for that

invalidity benefit! We needed the money—my loss of earnings and the extra cost of special diet foods was stretching our finances to the limit.

But the allowance, though helpful, underlined the reality of my predicament. I was now officially an invalid. Every day became a struggle to survive the black despair which gripped me.

By the end of February I had to be admitted to the Psychiatric Unit again. I felt frightened and guilty at being admitted a second time. How long would it be for? I'd spent six months of my life in limbo on this ward. Surely I wasn't going to have to go through all that again?

After the first week I was sent to the rehabilitation kitchen to learn how to cook with the limited foods I could tolerate. Soya milk, corn and rye were the staple ingredients.

Mavis, the occupational therapist in charge, made the task as pleasant as possible, always encouraging me with her warm smile. As we worked together to make a simple cake, I realised how weak I'd become. My hands were too feeble to beat the mixture, so I sat on the folding steps and she placed the bowl on a low stool. By holding the electric beater with both hands I managed to finish the job.

I'd made a cake, but I had to lie on my bed for the whole afternoon to recover.

Each day I battled in the kitchen to produce cakes and scones. Often I collapsed with sheer exhaustion and lay on the floor until I felt strong enough to get up and force myself to carry on.

'Chris, whatever's happened to you?' exclaimed my

friend Joan when she called unexpectedly to visit me at home. I'd been discharged from the Psychiatric Unit after only three weeks and was awaiting admission to Dr King's ward.

No wonder my friend was astonished at the change in me. Great black circles ringed my eyes and my muscles were thin and wasted. I sat hunched on the sofa, unable to hold my head up, gaunt and bent like an old woman.

Not only did she see the physical changes, but my personality had changed drastically since she had last spoken to me. I'd become a sour, morose creature, snapping violently at everybody.

'I know what it is,' she cried suddenly, with a flash of inspiration. 'You must have become allergic to another food. I've seen patients like you at the allergy clinic I go to.'

I was so awful to live with that Peter, rather than wait any longer for a bed to become available on Dr King's ward, made an appointment for me to see a homeopath in Liverpool.

Dr Radford's house was enormous, lavishly furnished with antiques and beautiful Indian carpets. A small, slim man, he greeted me in a consulting room the size of a ballroom. Large maps of bodies covered in acupuncture points hung against the walls.

The doctor was dwarfed by his massive, leather-topped desk. Despite his lack of physical stature he possessed a strong, almost charismatic, personality.

'Two kinds of people come to consult me,' he confided, 'those who are interested in the unusual and those who are truly desperate.'

It was obvious which category I was in! He discovererd that I'd become allergic to yeast and we left his office clutching a long list of foods to be avoided.

It seemed that the more the doctors tried to help me, the more foods they discovered I was allergic to. And it wasn't just food. There were hidden dangers such as the dust in the air and my own natural body yeasts. Eventually I even needed to filter all the chlorine out of the water I used for cooking or drinking.

I learned a great deal about how to manage such a complicated illness from the M.E. Society. Because the disease was incurable and little or no research was being funded by the National Health Service, our only hope of a cure was to organise ourselves into a support group and start raising funds, with the help of our families and friends. A highly qualified specialist was employed to give advice and co-ordinate the society's own research programme.

Peter and I went down by train to the society's annual general meeting in London. The hall was filled with ghastly, pale people, collapsed in their seats, many wearing surgical collars to support their drooping heads.

Several doctors spoke at length during the day but their message could have been summed up in one sentence: 'We are searching for a needle in a haystack.'

The atmosphere was deadly. Depression lay like a lead weight in my heart as I realised that in this room was the sum total of all knowledge about this terrible disease which had so cruelly brought my life to a standstill. *And nobody had any answers.*

Dr King had gently tried to show me this the last time I was admitted to his ward, when I'd asked him about the possibility of returning to work.

'I've had a letter from the hospital secretary,' I'd told him when he came to discuss the results of the latest round of tests. 'She needs to know when I'll be able to go back to work, otherwise they'll have to readvertise my job.'

He sat down on the end of my bed. 'I hope to get you better than you are now,' he said. 'But I don't realistically ever see you working again.'

I was shattered. *Never* work again? I felt that my life had ended. I loved my work. Surely I'd be able to go back one day?

He shook his head. 'It isn't fair to expect them to keep your job open for ever,' he said. 'I think you should write and tell them to give it to someone else.'

9

Wheelchair holiday

It took me exactly ten minutes to decide what I was going to do with the rest of my life.

After Dr King had left me I looked honestly at the sort of job I could do if, like some M.E. patients, I became too weak to walk at all. I'd lost my physical strength, it was true, which ruled out working as a physiotherapist, but I still had twenty years' experience in rehabilitation. I had my skill as an artist and my qualifications in adult education, but, most of all, I enjoyed helping people.

I thought of the time I'd spent in so many hospitals, both as a member of staff and as a patient, and suddenly I knew what I wanted to do. I would train as an art therapist! I wrote immediately to a college in Manchester for information about their training courses. In the meantime I had to find some way of surviving on a day-to-day basis.

Dr King's allergy tests had shown that there were only five foods left to which I was definitely not allergic.

'How on earth can I live on this?' I wondered, looking at the scrap of paper on which my short list was written: potatoes, oats, sugar, apples and chicken or eggs. This was all I had left to survive on. Even comforting cups of tea and coffee were now a thing of the past. I would have to get used to herbal teas instead.

'It's impossible!' I said bitterly. 'I can't even eat very much of these foods or I'll become allergic to them, too.'

Dr King made up a cocktail of allergens into a drug which I injected myself with every other day, in the hope that continued exposure to tiny amounts of the foods which made me ill would help build up my resistance to them.

I came home from the hospital exhausted and frazzled by the seemingly endless list of restrictions. Having been used to living such a full and busy life, I hated being so weak, looking such a wreck and needing so much care and attention. I just wanted to be *normal* again!

As we walked through our front door the phone was ringing. It was Joan, just back from a visit to her allergy clinic and feeling full of enthusiasm.

'I'm thinking of cooking a special dinner,' she announced, 'using only permitted foods. Would you like to come?'

'Well, I can only eat five different things now,' I warned her.

'No problem,' she said airily. 'Tell me what they are and we'll have them.' So, eagerly we accepted.

Joan's house overlooked the River Dee. A vast picture-window framed a magnificent cloud formation over the Welsh hills and we relaxed on the long sofa sipping herbal tea, gazing out over this beautiful view and feeling drowsily content after a delicious meal.

Joan, though, was full of suppressed excitement.

'What's the matter?' I asked her.

'I think I've found something that will help you,' she told me eagerly. 'I met a woman at the clinic who was using a pendulum to test her food before eating it.'

'What do you mean?'

'It's called dowsing,' she explained. 'Your body's tolerance to food alters considerably from day to day—even between morning and night. This lady could test her food with the pendulum to find out if it would harm her. It's based on the same principle as water-divining.'

We were fascinated. We all made little pendulums from tapestry needles and lengths of cotton thread and crowded into the kitchen to see if it worked. As I held the needle over a piece of food, like magic the needle began to swing. My hand was quite still, but the needle swung either from side to side or round and round, depending on whether the food was good for me or not.

I had no control over which way it would go; the needle seemed to have a life of its own. I tested some foods which I rarely ate and as most of these seemed to be OK I made a list of them. Thrilled at the thought of being able to supplement my diet in this way, I put the little pendulum into my purse and we said goodnight.

After that I always used it to test my food and Joan brought me a beautiful beechwood one which I used at home, blissfully unaware that the practice could ever be anything but helpful.

The M.E. Society wrote offering us a new diet which they claimed had helped people in Australia and New Zealand. It was called the Rotation Diet. Foods were divided up into different families, and only one family of food was eaten each day. This gave the body a break from that particular food for the rest of the week, so that it would, hopefully, cause less of an allergic reaction.

We were always ready to try anything new, but with only five foods and seven days in a week I was in trouble! Joan came to the rescue and together we worked out a rota using my five foods and a few unusual things like cashew nuts and arrowroot to bulk it out a bit.

My neighbour, Jane, who lived across the road, turned out to be a brilliantly inventive cook and she experimented with my pitifully limited supply of ingredients, producing cakes, scones and biscuits from potato or sago flour. She kept appearing at the door with a little pile of her latest creations on a plate, always with the recipe written out to go with it.

Joan found useful recipes from her allergy clinic, too, so together we coped. I know I couldn't have managed without their help.

Gradually, Peter and I built our lives around this strange new routine, and got so used to it that we began to think we might risk planning a family holiday. The National Women's Register ran a house-exchange scheme and we arranged to go to a cottage in Gloucestershire, taking my mother with us.

The cottage was an old, double-fronted house at the end of an overgrown lane. The plumbing was erratic, with taps which stopped flowing at the most inconvenient times, and the television could only be turned on with a pair of pliers. But the garden was lovely, with sunny lawns, shady apple trees and a friendly black cat.

Our main problem was the hills. I could barely walk any distance at all so, rather than spend the whole holiday confined to the garden, we had brought a wheelchair with us. Peter, though hard-pressed, was inexhaustible, pushing me up and down the steep roads in the town.

I'll never forget the first time we used the chair. My mother stood beside me as I climbed in, trying not to show her feelings and pretending to be quite unmoved by the sight.

Peter's lack of experience in handling the wheelchair was demonstrated as we struck the first kerb. I was jack-knifed violently forwards, almost landing on the pavement. I hung on tightly as he bashed and slammed his way across the side roads until his technique gradually improved.

The streets were crowded with people, pushing and hurrying, pressing in on us tightly. All at once the dreadful tide of their pity hit me as I sat in the chair. Some smiled, others looked away. I felt as though I wasn't a normal forty-year-old woman any more. I was an unacceptable object of sympathy in a wheelchair.

When we reached the shops where I'd wanted to get out and look around, I froze, overcome with embarrassment. 'I can't get out of this and start walking about,' I muttered to Peter. 'What will people think if they suddenly see me start walking?'

'Don't worry about them—we're here to enjoy ourselves,' he insisted. But I refused to budge, so we turned around and made our way home again.

'I'm not going to be beaten,' I decided, once back within

the safety of our cottage. 'Tomorrow, when we go out,
I'm going to get in and out of that chair as I please.'

The next day we went to Slimbridge Wildfowl
Sanctuary. As we went through the entrance, a deputation
of forty-odd ducks came waddling to meet us. The sun
shone brightly in a perfect summer sky; swathes of
glorious wild flowers surrounded the wildlife pools, their
tiny petals scattering colour through the rich green rushes.

Wherever we went beautiful birds came and fed from
our hands. It was a day of total happiness.

'This is wonderful, Peter,' I cried, as we sat eating our
picnic lunch beside a lake, watching the swans. 'I'm so
glad we came. I could never have plucked up the courage
to come away on holiday if Dr Kennedy hadn't spent
so much time with me.'

Dr Kennedy, the new registrar at the Psychiatric Unit
which I still attended for weekly therapy as an outpatient,
was a man who somehow made me believe the very best
about myself. Having persuaded me that I really could
cope with a week away from the security of home, he
was now working on giving me confidence in my ability
to manage the art therapy course which was due to start
in the autumn.

We roamed around the bird sanctuary for the rest of
the day, enjoying a rare oasis of contentment in our barren
lives, only reluctantly making our way back to the cottage
when dusk fell.

Our next outing was to the standing stones at Avebury,
where we were going on the recommendation of Dr
Radford, the homeopath. I'd been eagerly looking forward

to seeing them. The stone circles were set around and amid the quaint old village and its surrounding bun-shaped hills.

As we got out of the car a violent gust of scorching wind hit us, bowling all our belongings away across the grass.

Braced against the wind and perspiring in the intense heat, we set off to look for a picnic spot, Peter weaving the wheelchair in and out through the languid sheep grazing among the stones. We settled down in the lee of a monstrous stone and ate our lunch, then, overcome by the effort and swamped by a sense of desolation, I lay down on the grass and cried.

Determined not to spoil the day, I climbed back into the wheelchair and Peter pushed me back towards the village. Nearing a group of stones known as The Cove, we came across some people dowsing with huge, black pendulums.

'Why are you dowsing?' Peter asked them.

'This is a healing stone,' a tall Swiss man answered. Then, seeing me in the wheelchair, he invited us to join them. We all gathered around a gigantic, fat stone and he held his pendulum against my back. 'The energy level in your spine is very low,' he informed me, 'and in your neck it's almost non-existent.'

Testing the fat stone with his pendulum, he pointed to a particular spot and told me to lean against it. Amazingly, I felt energy flowing through my body. The depression lifted and we went on our way, thanking them profusely.

'Fancy finding a healing stone,' I said, delighted to be feeling better again. 'Dowsing really works, doesn't it?'

But despite appearing to help at the time, its effect soon wore off. When we got back home from our holiday I was as ill and depressed as ever.

'I'm never going to get better,' I told myself, staring miserably into the washing-up water as I stood at the kitchen sink, trying to tidy things a bit. 'I'm no good to Peter or to Sally. I'm not living any sort of real life. The only possible use there is left for me is to donate my body for spare-part surgery.'

Common sense told me that no surgeon would consider killing off one patient to use their organs to save the life of another, but I did wonder if there was any way I could commit suicide and yet donate my body to be of use to someone else.

'Exit, the Euthanasia Society, would know,' I thought. 'I'm going to get in touch with them.'

10

Caring friends

'I've had a phone call from an old friend of yours,' my mother informed me over the telephone early one Saturday morning. 'Do you remember Joy Tyler?'

'You mean the girl who lived across the road from us when I was about ten?' I asked incredulously. 'How on earth did she get in touch?'

'Remember the sponsored ramble the Women's Institute held to raise money for the M.E. Society's research programme?'

Of course I remembered the ramble. Of the eight ladies who had taken part, only one was under sixty and four others were over seventy. During their ten-mile walk they had stopped off to pose for a photograph outside a cafe. When I saw the beaming row of smiling faces, posing beneath the cafe's hanging baskets, I felt quite overcome with emotion. They were so old, yet they'd walked all those miles for me, raising £208 to help towards finding a cure.

Due to the ramblers' zeal in collecting the money, practically everybody in the village had heard about myalgic encephalomyelitis. Its awesomeness was enhanced by the fact that nobody could pronounce it properly!

Mother went on: 'Joy met your friend Wendy, and Wendy told her you were very ill with the disease.'

'So what did Joy want?' I asked, curious to know what had prompted her to get in touch after all these years.

'It seems she's one of these "born again" Christians now,' said Mother. 'She says God has told her he can heal you. I don't suppose you'd want to see her, would you?'

'Oh, no,' I thought, 'I don't want anything to do with a religious nut!'

Then I felt mean. Just like everyone else who had heard of my illness, this kind woman was offering help in her own way. I couldn't reject her. 'Oh, all right. I'd better see her,' I said, and we rang off.

Joy arrived half an hour later. She bounced into the house and threw her arms around me. Peter took one look and disappeared into the kitchen. Ten minutes later he went out shopping, leaving me alone with this vibrant woman who seemed to fill the whole house with happiness. I'd never met anyone like her before.

'God has been so good to me,' she told me. 'My marriage was virtually on the rocks before I became a Christian. I was going to take my two children and leave my husband.'

'What happened?' I wondered, interested now, though I'd meant to get rid of her as soon as possible.

'We were desperate,' she went on, 'until we went along to a charismatic church. Then God changed us and we fell in love all over again.'

I didn't know what she was talking about. I'd never heard of a charismatic church, but I sat quietly and listened as she told me how, only two weeks ago, she had been healed of a painful frozen shoulder at a meeting in Wales.

Peter came back, dragging the basket on wheels laden with our shopping. He was actually whistling! I hadn't heard him whistle for a long time. Joy jumped up and put both her hands on my head and began to pray for me. Then she asked if we would go to a meeting being held that night by a church in Liverpool.

'We couldn't possibly go,' Peter explained. 'Chris can't sit up for more than a few minutes. She'd need a special padded chair to support her back and head.'

I agreed. It was one thing to collapse on the floor at the Psychiatric Unit but quite another during a public meeting.

'Ring me if you change your mind,' said Joy brightly before she left.

Throughout the rest of the day we felt uneasy and disturbed by Joy's visit, until finally, about an hour before the meeting was due to start, we decided to go.

'I don't care if I do end up lying on the floor,' I declared. 'I might as well be ill there as at home.' It would be uncomfortable and embarrassing, but I was willing to try anything to get better.

There were crowds of people at the meeting—it was much bigger than anything we'd imagined. Teenagers wearing jeans and sweaters crammed the hall, singing and shouting their love for Jesus. They waved their hands in the air and danced up and down the aisles. The leaders of the church, mostly middle-aged (and some with more than a little middle-age spread) stood on the platform, joining in the dancing and shouting with gusto.

'I've never seen anything like this in my life,' I said to Joy in astonishment, but she just grinned and pointed to a man on the platform dressed in a white tuxedo jacket which, with his fair hair, made him look like my idea of an angel.

'He's our church leader,' she told me proudly.

I tried to stand up and join in the clapping and singing but I was too exhausted to do anything for more than a few moments. Too tired to sit up any longer, I lay across Peter's lap and rested as the meeting went on. I'd dozed off when one of the leaders came forward to the microphone to speak.

'There's a lady here who has been very ill for about two years,' he announced. 'She also has severe depression. If you'd like to come out to the front we'll pray with you.'

How on earth could he have known?

'That's you,' cried Joy excitedly. 'Go on out and let them pray for you.'

But I stayed rooted to the spot. No way was I going to show myself up in front of all those people!

'No, I'll stay here with you,' I said. Joy put her arm around me and prayed, but I didn't feel any different.

The next morning, the amazing meeting of the night before seemed unreal in the cold light of day. The people there had obviously been on very familiar terms with God and it was frightening and strange for us, who had only ever been to traditional church services. We only knew God as a remote figure, to be worshipped in a restrained, typically British, way, so we pushed the experience to the back of our minds.

At the Psychiatric Unit, Dr Kennedy informed us that he was leaving to work in a prison. It was a tremendous blow, but a great tribute to the work he had done with me that I was able to accept the news without breaking down.

He spent our last therapy session building into me the confidence I needed to face my interview for a place on the art therapy training course. Before the interview, Peter drove me to the college in Manchester to make sure I'd be able to walk the distance from the station where I would arrive by train each morning. We were relieved to find it wasn't very far.

I was interviewed by two stern middle-aged ladies. One wanted me, the other obviously didn't, but I was accepted and I returned home triumphant. And so began my bizarre double life: one day each week learning how to teach pyschiatric patients as an art therapist, another day attending a Psychiatric Unit as a patient.

Sticking to the course was hard going when I felt ill or tired, but despite the effort it required I looked forward to it. It was my only hope for the future; everything seemed to hang on my continued presence and success at the college.

Getting there by train was a major operation. Rising before dawn, I would leave home while it was still dark, drive my car to Chester station, then board the train to Manchester. Most mornings it was almost empty when it left Chester so I would lie on the long seats and rest until crowds of noisy schoolchildren joined us. After that

I would prop myself up in a corner for the rest of the way.

'Have you had your injection?' Peter would ask before I left home. 'Have you got your medicine and your food for the day?' We had rearranged my rotation diet so that potatoes were eaten on Fridays and I could join the girls in the canteen at lunchtime for a plate of chips cooked in vegetable oil. My other food aroused curiosity.

'What on earth are you eating?' they asked, eyeing the dried up bits and pieces I kept nibbling throughout the day.

'It's my special diet food,' I told them. 'I have to eat every two hours or I simply collapse.'

I always arrived at the college before anyone else and immediately went to drag my special chair from the library into the lecture room. It had a padded back and seat, which was vital if I was to be able to sit through a whole day's lectures. My muscles were now so wasted that my protruding bones pinched the skin into painful bruises if I sat on an ordinary hard chair.

Jules, the first lecturer, would stroll in a little later, puffing casually on his pipe, then one by one the rest of the group would trickle sleepily in to start the day. It irritated me to see the scant importance they gave to their studies when it cost me so much to be there.

To me, that course meant the difference between life and death. I needed a reason for living, some hope of fulfilment in my life; without that I simply didn't want to carry on enduring such a painful struggle for survival.

The terrifying spectre of a cabbage-like existence in a wheelchair haunted me day and night—so much so that I had secretly been to the Citizens Advice Bureau to ask

for the address of Exit, the Euthanasia Society. I had felt
sure that, after contacting them, I would find peace in
death and an end to our family's misery.

But I hadn't bargained on finding an unexpected ally,
another champion fighting for my cause. The Citizens
Advice Bureau was housed in a rather grand old house
at the far side of the park. Posters lined the walls of the
entrance hall offering impartial advice on any subject from
what to do if a nuclear bomb dropped to the venue of
the local mother and toddler group.

Tea was being made when I arrived, so I had to wait
until a small middle-aged lady came along to lead me into
a sunny back room overlooking a tangled garden. In a
business-like manner I explained what I'd come for.

'Why do you want this address?' she asked suspiciously,
as if she thought I was planning to do away with all my
rich relatives. By the time I'd finished telling her why
I needed it she was on my side. She gave me a telephone
number and told me to ring any time, day or night. I
left the building without the address I'd come for, but
wrapped in a warm glow from the love and kindness
she had shown.

My days at the Psychiatric Unit were now spent, not
in hard-hitting therapy sessions as they had been with
Dr Kennedy, but in the hospital day centre, engraving
pewter with the chronically ill patients. I was shocked
when the ward sister told me to join them.

'But that's for the really hopeless cases,' I cried. 'How
will I get better if I'm not part of the therapy group?'

'The group is for limited numbers of patients,' she

explained. 'You've been in the group for a year now and there are other people waiting for a place.'

Day by day my frustration increased until finally I could bear it no longer. Spotting Dr Hesketh, a young psychiatrist who was a new member of staff, walking along the corridor, I grabbed the front of his white coat. 'Help me, please,' I wept, hanging on to him. 'Please help me to get better, before I get any worse!'

Something in my desperation must have touched him, for instead of pushing me away he said gently, 'It's all right, I'll help you. I'll come and see you at the day hospital.'

After that we met every Tuesday in a tiny lounge and battled together to find an answer. He discovered I'd even become allergic to the five foods I had left to eat and my diet became more drab than ever.

He was young, clever and eager to help. But as the weeks went by I got sicker, thinner and more frantic, while he became more and more at a loss to know what to do. But at least he gave me hope. Each time I saw him he lifted me into life again for another week.

11

Satan in the poppyfield

'We're having another meeting tonight,' said Joy, ringing me early one Saturday morning in November. 'It's called a Celebration Evening. Would you like to come?'

I hadn't thought much about the meeting we'd been to before, but as soon as Joy invited us I knew I wanted to go with her again.

'I'll get there early and save you a couple of seats,' she offered, 'then you won't have to sit upright for any longer than necessary.'

It was a new concept for us, saving seats at church in case you couldn't all get in—certainly none of the churches we'd ever been to before had had such a problem. But sure enough, when we arrived, the meeting room was full to bursting point and stewards were directing people to seats in an overflow hall where they could listen to the meeting through loudspeakers.

We found Joy valiantly defending our seats and sat down beside her and her husband, Derek, just as the musicians began to play. The pianist was quite spectacular, playing lively songs in a jazzy, modern style. I looked around at the faces of those around me, shining with

happiness as they sang with all their heart songs of praise
to God. Sitting back in my chair I let it all flow around me.

On the platform were the men in suits again, and there
was Dave, the angel in the tuxedo jacket. Everyone was
clapping and dancing. The meeting was full of triumph.
God was there—I couldn't doubt it.

As we watched, one of the leaders stepped forward to the
microphone and looked around at the congregation, who
stood expectantly, waiting to hear what he had to say.

'There is a lady here,' he announced, 'who is suffering
from severe depression. God wants to heal you. Just come
forward to the platform and we'll pray for you.'

It had happened again! I sat uncertainly in my seat,
wondering if the lady concerned was me, but somehow
I didn't think it was. A few moments later, a short, plump
lady made her way down the aisle to the front of the
meeting, tears openly pouring down her cheeks. I watched
sceptically as the man who had spoken stepped down
from the platform to meet her, laid his hands on her head
and prayed with real compassion for God to heal her of
the terrible depression which was destroying her life.

She was transformed before our eyes! The tears stopped,
the expression on her face showed clearly that the
depression had lifted, and in its place there came a peace
which radiated from her as she walked back to her seat.

'I'd like to see her again in a month's time,' I thought
cynically, all my medical training coming to the fore. But
somehow, deep inside, I knew she had been healed.

As the meeting went on my brain whirled, trying to
make sense of what I'd just witnessed. I had battled for

more than two years to conquer my depression. I'd had the very best treatment at the hospital; my family and friends had loved and cared for me; I'd pitted every ounce of strength and intelligence I possessed against this monster which gripped me—yet week by week I grew worse, not better.

I looked across at the lady who had gone forward for prayer. She seemed to glow with happiness. Oh, how I wished it could have been me!

'I've got to talk to that man,' I said urgently to Peter as the meeting ended. So he helped me push my way through the crowds until we reached the visiting speaker, a man named Bryn Jones.

'What do you want me to pray for?' he asked, as I stood before him.

'To be healed, like the other lady,' I should have said. But I didn't. I simply couldn't say the words. 'Please pray for my life to go in the right direction,' I mumbled. Placing his hands on the top of my head, he prayed exactly that, and Peter took me home.

'Chris, you're lacking in emotion!' declared the art therapy tutor at college that week. 'You need to use plenty of water in your painting to help express yourself more freely.'

Obediently, I reached for the water-pot and, selecting the red and green paints, began work on my favourite subject, a poppyfield, taking care to slosh the water about freely, as I'd been told. Suddenly, I found I had painted an enormous black figure, completely obliterating the poppies!

Oozing from the watery paper, there was no doubt in my mind who the figure was: it was Satan.

For somebody lacking in emotion, I moved fast! I rushed out of the room, along the corridor, down the stairs, through the front door and into the carpark.

'This is ridiculous,' I told myself firmly. 'It's just paint! Get back in there.'

Reluctantly, I made my way back up the stairs into the classroom. I slapped another piece of paper on the desk and began to work once more. Horror of horrors—there was Satan again, huge and black, with his great foot trying to kick me! I shot out of the building, right through the front gate and down the main road, shaking with fright and panting with the effort.

I knew I had to go back. We had instructions to keep all our therapy paintings—I had to write essays about them as part of my course work. So, slowly, I made my way back to the class, rolled up the hated paintings and took them home.

The following two art therapy days were disastrous. My paintings became more and more disturbed, the discussion sessions were full of tension and I began to feel persecuted by those who I knew were really dear friends.

Even Dr Hesketh was beginning to despair. My screams of fear were like claws digging into him.

'I feel so sorry for you, Chris,' he admitted. 'My own wife is a physiotherapist and pianist, just as you were. When I look at you I realise that it could have been her.'

He finally decided that in the New Year he would put

me on a powerful drug, one used sparingly by psychiatrists because of the ease with which patients became addicted to it and the violent hallucinations which accompanied its withdrawal. Dr Hesketh gave me a card with a long list of foods which must be avoided when taking the drug, a list which usually caused patients to gasp in horror at the thought of such a restricted diet.

I read through it. 'It makes no difference to me,' I said, gloomily. 'I can't eat any of these things anyway.'

To take this drug was, as far as I was concerned, equivalent to entering a no-man's-land between life and death. I was terrified by what I had seen happening to another patient treated with it, but I was so ill and mentally tormented that I agreed to the treatment. I was still willing to try anything that might make life a little easier.

With the coming of the new year something died inside me. I'd struggled for so long but now I felt I couldn't for one moment longer bear the mental and physical torture this wretched disease had inflicted upon me. I didn't care whether I lived or died—the misery just had to stop.

Reaching into my bedside drawer, I took out the bottles of pills kept there and shook some of each into my hand. There was no thought of suicide in my mind; I'd gone way beyond being methodical enough to try to kill myself. I just felt an overwhelming need to blot everything out. I swallowed the pills, then sleepily reached for the phone.

'Is that you, Sister?' I asked, my voice beginning to slur a little as the drugs began to take effect. 'It's Chris.

I . . . I can't stand it any more. I've taken some extra pills
. . . . I'm going to take some more whenever I wake up.'

The ward sister must have acted fast, for by the time
I'd replaced the phone, staggered downstairs and taken
another lot of pills, a community psychiatric nurse was
at the front door.

I lay in the armchair, dimly aware of him talking to
a doctor who arrived a few minutes later.

'How many pills did you take?' they asked. 'Have you
taken any more since you rang the ward?'

I didn't care. What did it matter how many I had taken?

I was admitted to the high dependency ward at the
Psychiatric Unit, where a kind young doctor examined
me. 'Why did you do it?' he asked. I lay drowsily in the
bed, trying to focus my eyes on his face. I couldn't answer
him.

'Was it because you just couldn't cope any more?' he
persisted.

I nodded briefly before finally falling over the edge of
consciousness into the oblivion I'd longed for.

Hours later, when I eventually woke up, I looked
around the tiny ward at my fellow patients. In the next
bed was Ruth—or, rather, what was left of Ruth. This
girl had poured petrol over herself and set it alight. She
had survived but was one horrific mass of scars.

Opposite was Grace, a girl suffering from a combination
of anorexia and religious mania. She deprived herself of
food on the pretext of fasting and was now close to death.

Later in the day Dr Hesketh came to visit and transferred
me back to the ward I'd been on before. Three times I'd

been admitted to the same ward. How far away it now seemed when I'd arrived for the first time, honestly believing that after a three-week stay I would be cured and ready to start life again! Two years later I was back where I'd started.

The most urgent matter was my food, for the overdose had weakened me and I was too ill to cook. Peter took the bags of grain to Joan's house and she quickly made up some food for me and he brought it along in a basket.

When he arrived, Dr Hesketh called him into the office for a long talk.

'I'm afraid we don't hold out any hope of your wife's condition improving, Mr Youngman,' he said. 'There's really nothing more we can do.'

'But we can't carry on like this!' Peter insisted, at the end of his tether with the strain of coping with my illness and the added shock of my taking an overdose.

'The only thing I can suggest,' offered the doctor sympathetically, 'is for you to have her at home until you feel you can't cope any longer, then we'll readmit her for a couple of weeks to give you a chance to rest.'

What a humiliating vision of the future it presented! I, who had lived a full and useful life, to be passed back and forth like a hot potato, a burden to everybody. I wept bitterly when Dr Hesketh broke the news to me.

'Good morning, Peter,' cried Joy, full of good cheer when she rang him a few days later. 'We're having another Celebration Evening in Chester. Would you and Chris like to come?'

'No, we wouldn't!' snapped Peter. 'What is there to

celebrate? Chris is in hospital again. She took an overdose of drugs.'

Joy appeared at the Psychiatric Unit, bursting into a ward full of visitors, and quickly spotted me propped up in a geriatric chair.

She got straight down to business. 'Well, what about asking Jesus into your life then? He's keen to get to work on you, you know, but he won't force himself upon you. You need to pray and invite him.' She totally ignored the curious gaze of the other visitors crowding into the lounge.

I didn't care either. I'd completely lost interest in my life and nothing mattered to me at all.

'All right, go ahead,' I said, and mechanically repeated a prayer, word for word, after her. I felt no different at all but Joy was exultant. She flung her arms around me and squashed me in a great bear-hug.

When she let go, I looked up and saw my friend, Elsa, from the Heswall Women's Register, standing in the doorway holding a bunch of flowers, watching us in astonishment.

12

The day of humiliation

Elsa had come to take me home. But when her car pulled up outside our front door I knew I couldn't do it.

I simply couldn't face walking into the empty house and spending the day alone there, waiting until Peter and Sally came home. I would rather go straight in and take another lot of pills, for death held no fear for me compared with the terror of being left alone.

Elsa was on her way to a meeting of the Women's Register knitting circle, little dreaming that as soon as she dropped me off I intended to kill myself. Then I thought of how she would feel when she heard the news. Though these days nobody could accurately predict what I would do next, I knew she would blame herself.

'Please take me with you to Annette's house, Elsa,' I asked. Obligingly, she took me along and I lay huddled in an armchair, withdrawn and silent, while they knitted and chatted together.

As they packed up their work at lunchtime, Annette quietly handed me a sheet of notepaper with eight names and telephone numbers written on it. 'Take this, Chris,' she said, 'and pin it up next to your phone. If you ever feel suicidal again, ring any of us and we'll come round straightaway.'

Elsa drove me home and I lay on the sofa for a little while, covered with a knitted patchwork blanket, until Peter and Sally came home for tea.

Peter looked strained and worn out, tired beyond belief. He had finally accepted that I was dying, that if I didn't succeed in killing myself first, the ridiculous diet would finish me off. For my sake, he hoped I wouldn't suffer much longer. For himself, he knew he'd reached the end of his ability to cope.

While I'd been recovering in hospital Peter had received a phone call from Joy, offering to have me to stay with them for a few days.

'Thank you, Joy, but no,' he'd replied firmly, convinced that she had no idea what was involved in caring for me, and concerned about the strain it would place on her husband and three children. But now he changed his mind and rang her back, gratefully accepting the offer.

'You're going to stay with Joy tomorrow,' he informed me, having made the arrangements.

'I'm not,' I declared, horrified at the idea of being ill in someone else's home—especially one full of noisy children.

'Chris, you've *got* to go,' he insisted, almost beside himself with desperation. 'I just can't manage any longer. You either go to Joy's or go back to the hospital.'

Rebelliously I packed my belongings: a few clothes and an enormous basket of drugs, special foods, the water-filter and my dowsing needle.

In contrast to what I'd been expecting, Joy's home was

full of peace. The children, Philip, Isobel and Anna, were out at school all day, and I would lie quietly on the sofa while Joy read psalms to me and sang beautifully.

One by one, the children would come home, always curious at the sight of their sick visitor but, having been warned how ill I was, careful not to overwhelm me with noise or attention. Then Derek would arrive and take his place at the head of the table, trying to hide his disgust at the pile of green slime which was my main meal for the day.

After three days the suicidal terror had gone and I went home to Peter for the weekend. He was still edgy, nervous of leaving me and obviously relieved when Tuesday arrived and he could take me back to the hospital for the day. The headmaster of the school where he taught was sympathetic and understanding about the difficulties he faced and agreed that Peter could go in late after he'd seen me safely into the hospital's care.

Driving along the leafy, tree-lined avenues, he seemed tense and distracted. Then suddenly he slammed on the brakes, pulled the car into the side of the road and burst into tears. His shoulders heaved and shook as he sobbed and sobbed, on and on as if he would never stop.

I sat and watched him, powerless to help or offer any crumb of hope or comfort. I couldn't believe it was happening. Peter, my calm husband who had stood by me through all these hell-like years was breaking up in front of my eyes!

Eventually he started up the car again, delivered me to the hospital ward and went on to school, where the children racketed around him, unchecked, all day. Friends who saw him were shocked at the sight of his white, drawn face. 'He looks as if he's on the edge of a nervous breakdown,' they whispered.

I crouched in a corner of the day ward, propping up my aching head, wishing there was some way I could find relief from the strain of trying to support it. 'Maybe the staff have made a decision about the neck support collar I asked for,' I wondered, heaving myself with tremendous effort on to my feet.

I knocked at the office door and asked the nurse in charge about it.

'No dear, we don't really think it would help much,' she replied casually, obviously not realising how painful my neck was. 'Can you pop along to your therapy group now, please?'

I felt angry—very angry. My life was such misery. Surely anything which could offer even the slightest relief should be tried, not dismissed so easily. I determined there and then to get a collar, no matter how much fuss I had to make.

After lunch I saw my chance. I was resting in the hall on the settee when Dr Hesketh came along, wearing his anorak, ready to go home and start his holidays. Time and time again this poor man had taken his driving test and failed, so here he was, sheltering from the pouring rain, waiting for his taxi to arrive.

'Have you done anything about getting the neck collar I need?' I asked hopefully.

'Well, no,' he admitted. 'Why not go and have a chat

with the physiotherapist about it?'

'I already have,' I wailed in frustration, 'and she told me to have a chat with you!' He edged nearer the doors and peered out eagerly through the streaming glass, preparing to escape as soon as the taxi arrived to rescue him.

Desperate and furious, I grabbed him by the front of his anorak and screamed at the top of my voice.

'If you'd take the trouble to examine my neck you'd see that my muscles are too wasted to support my head,' I yelled, ignoring the crowd of inquisitive patients flooding into the hallway on their way back from lunch.

'Look at me!' I shouted. 'Look at my neck! There should be thick muscle tissue there—but instead it's full of hollows. Have you never studied anatomy?'

Puce-faced, Dr Hesketh shook himself free and rushed through the entrance doors to stand outside in the rain, preferring a good soaking to my fearsome company.

Trembling with fury and wretched with frustration, I turned my back on the soggy figure outside the doors and made my way upstairs. I was determined not to be beaten. I would see the physiotherapist again.

I knew her well. She had been a fellow-student at the physiotherapy training college and, later, a close colleague on the Stroke Unit. But our present roles divided us like east and west.

I sank on to her couch and my friend swivelled in her chair to face me. 'Jenny, I've just got to have that neck collar,' I said miserably.

'I can't give you one,' was her cool reply. 'I've written

to the consultant of the M.E. Society in London, and you'll have to wait until he writes back with his advice.'

But I couldn't wait. I could be dead by the time he got round to answering. I needed help now! Oh, how could I make her understand?

'Jenny, I don't believe you'd deliberately leave a patient to suffer unnecessary pain,' I begged, hating myself for putting her in such a difficult position. 'Please help me.'

She wasn't enjoying the interview either.

'Chris, it's *because* your neck is so weak that I don't know if a collar will help or harm you,' she said. 'There are no muscles covering the blood vessels in your shoulders. The pressure of the collar could make things even more painful for you.'

Nevertheless she reluctantly went to the store cupboard, brought out a selection of collars and tried each one on me in turn. She was right, they were all very uncomfortable, but she gave me the one that fitted best.

'Only wear it for short periods of time, when the pain in your neck is really unbearable,' she advised.

I left, relieved to have finally got the collar but humiliated at the scene I'd had to cause.

Grovelling to a colleague was the final indignity!

13

The day of miracles

The sloppy mass of grey and yellow food lay in an unappetising heap on my plate.

'Yuck!' said Anna, Joy and Derek's eight-year-old daughter, pulling a face. 'How can you eat such horrible dinner, Auntie Chris?'

The rest of the family were equally uninhibited about expressing their opinion of my ghastly concoction, turning up their noses in disgust as they tucked into their meat and vegetables.

This was my second visit to stay in their home. The ice had now been well and truly broken and, as they accepted me into their family, the polite, general conversation was abandoned. I had lived with my diet for so long that neither Peter nor Sally ever bothered to comment on it any more, but the thought of eating such bland, uninteresting food clearly appalled this family.

'I'm going to a prayer meeting in Chester tonight,' young Philip informed me meaningfully, 'and we're all going to pray for you.'

I lay on the sofa watching television, with Anna and Isobel wedged in around me. Isobel was trying to draw a shoe for her art homework.

'I keep getting it wrong,' she muttered despairingly,

screwing up the paper and throwing it in the bin. 'You were an artist, Chris. Could you help me, please?'

I struggled into a sitting position and tried to show her how to draw the shoe, but my attempt was worse than hers. Had I ever really sold my work to shops in Covent Garden?

I lay awake all that night, listening to Anna's intermittent cough and knitting a friend's sweater to pass the time. Knitting was one of the few skills I'd managed to hang on to. Whenever I felt well enough to sit up and concentrate, I would knit for a while. Sometimes I designed my own sweaters, and my friends and the staff and patients at the Psychiatric Unit often asked me to knit for them. They bought the wool and I charged them about £10 for my work. I had quite a little business going!

I woke the next morning with a head fit to burst, so when Joy came bouncing into the bedroom with her big smile I felt I couldn't bear to see anyone so full of life and happiness when I felt like death.

'How are you this morning?' she inquired.

'Rotten,' I declared, with venom in my voice. 'I hate everybody.'

'Everybody?' she asked, without batting an eyelid.

'Yes, everybody,' I insisted. 'Peter, Sally, my mother, the doctors—I hate them. They've all failed me.'

Even though it was me who was speaking, I could hardly believe what I was hearing. How could I say such awful things about the people I loved and who had stuck by me when I was so difficult to live with?

But it was as if a dam had broken inside me. Torrents

of words poured out in an uncontrollable tidal wave of hate, bitterness and resentment, surging and flooding over me until I didn't know what I was saying anymore. Joy stood by and listened but I didn't care. I raged on and on.

'And another thing!' I stormed, finally. 'My job in the Rehabilitation Unit meant everything to me. No matter what happens I'll never get over losing that. It's like . . . like being bereaved!'

Exhausted, I collapsed back into the bed and huddled down as far as I could go, miserably conscious of Joy still standing there. What must she think of me?

'This is wonderful!' she crowed, leaping into the air in triumph. 'You can repent of all this! You can give it all to God. I'll get my friend to come and we'll pray for you.'

'This woman is a complete nut!' I thought, as she rushed excitedly down the stairs to the phone before going out to take Anna to school.

'Liz is coming in about half an hour,' she announced when she got back. 'You might remember her, she's got multiple sclerosis.'

Multiple sclerosis. Well, God hadn't healed her, had he!

I sat on the bed, my heart in my boots, and hoped she wouldn't come. But before long the little blue invalid car was parked in the drive. I could hear the two of them downstairs in the lounge, praying together like a pair of twittering birds, so I stayed firmly put until Joy came to fetch me.

With a sigh of resignation I made my way downstairs. I sat on one end of the sofa and Joy perched on the other.

Liz sat beside me in an armchair—an invalid waiting to pray for another invalid. Yet she looked more like Joy than like me. She had that same shine on her face, that look of inner peace which, tantalisingly, I could see but had never known.

Joy got straight down to business.

'Chris, all that hatred you were feeling this morning is poisoning your life,' she said. 'If you want him to, God can change your life—give you a new start.'

'I could certainly do with one,' I thought. My life was a disaster.

'But before you can have a new life,' Joy went on, 'you have to sort out the old one. You see, although God is kind and loving, he's also holy and he can't have anything to do with us while we're still messed up with the wrong things we've done.

'That's why Jesus died on the cross. He took your punishment so that God could forgive you for all that hatred. You can have a new life, but first you need to ask God to forgive you for hating those people—and for any other wrong things you've done.'

I had never heard anything like it. But what a marvellous deal!

So I threw myself into it with all the energy I could muster, delving into the past, raking up anything I could think of which might have offended God so that I could have this wonderful new start. Then I prayed, asking his forgiveness for it all, not caring that Joy and Liz overheard me confessing all the personal details. I just wanted to do the job properly.

'I think that's everything,' I said, eventually.

'What about your Rehabilitation Unit?' asked Joy.

I thought for a moment. Suddenly, I felt overwhelmed with generosity towards God. After all, he was offering me so much—a brand new life. I decided to hand over my job on the unit to God. It had meant everything to me, it was the best thing I had ever achieved, so I made a present of it to him, along with the rest of my life. He could have the lot!

I abandoned everything—all my hopes and ambitions, my dreams and disappointments. Like taking a leap in the dark from a cliff-top—and trusting that someone would be there to catch me—I handed it all over to him.

The moment I did it things began to happen.

Throughout the whole of my illness I'd had a machine-like noise inside my head, a buzzing something like interference on a television set or the distant sound of a pneumatic drill. Trying to hear what people were saying to me through this noise was often such an effort that I gave up and withdrew into my shell rather than go on struggling to understand.

Now, the noise had completely gone, switched off instantly as if someone had pulled out the plug. The relief was indescribable! My blurred vision cleared, and my muffled ears opened as easily as if someone had come along and taken out a pair of earplugs.

Then, like a great plant being uprooted, taproot and all, the depression tore out of my body and seemed to disappear up into the ceiling.

I was healed! No scepticism this time. I was healed and

I knew it!

Then, like a mighty wind, came the presence of God, rushing inside me, filling me to overflowing with love and joy and peace of such intensity that I felt on fire with the glory of it.

Liz and Joy sat speechless, watching my glowing face. I was speechless, too, in a state of utter bliss. Liz left and I lay on the sofa all afternoon, wrapped in a cocoon of peace, feeling totally well for the first time in almost three years.

One by one, as the family arrived home, they were brought into the lounge to behold the miracle. I just lay there, grinning at everybody, enjoying their astonishment but too overwhelmed by the experience to say very much.

The next day, Joy and Derek took me home to Peter. Smirking like satisfied cats, they stood beside me in the hall and watched his expression as they explained what had happened.

Incredulity, amazement and hope chased each other across his face as he gazed at me. I knew what he was seeing. The haunted look had gone, my sunken face was alive again. Physically, I was still weak and wasted, but I radiated that something extra we had seen in the people at the church in Chester.

'Thank you,' gasped Peter, shaking Derek and Joy by the hand, struggling to hide the emotion which welled up inside and threatened to overcome him. 'Thank you so much!'

They left us alone and we sat together, talking excitedly about what this strange development would mean to us.

Oh, the joy of being able to hold a sensible, positive conversation again! We talked on and on.

'Hey, I'd better get you some tea,' said Peter, suddenly noticing the time. He went into the kitchen and I sat back on the hated sofa where I had spent so much time, tossed aside the patchwork blanket which had covered me when I lay in pain and despair, and revelled in the thought that I need never lie there again unless I really wanted to.

Peter boiled up some of my green slime and threw a few sausages into a frying-pan for himself.

Suddenly, the realisation of what had happened hit him. I was healed! The nightmare was over. The wife he had known and loved had seemed to die long ago, lost as irretrievably as if I really had died. He had suffered the same trauma and grief that any widower would go through, all the time bracing himself for the final blow of bereavement, when he really would lose me for ever. Now I was back with that old sparkle in my eyes, as if the last three years had never been.

I wasn't going to die. I was going to live—really live. The whole family was released from the prison of misery in which my illness had trapped us.

Great, fat tears rolled down his cheeks and plopped on to the cooker, blurring his eyes as he cooked the meal.

'It's over,' he whispered to himself, again and again. 'It really is over!'

14

'Whatever's happened to you?'

Sunday morning, in contrast to our usual weekend routine, we were up early, racing around to get dressed and have breakfast in good time. We were going to church!

We were bubbling over with excitement at the thought of it, remembering the Celebration Evenings, when anyone who arrived less than half an hour before starting time found the meeting room full to bursting point. We made sure we were out of the house and into the car in plenty of time.

When we arrived, we found the whole church had heard about the miracle of my healing. Complete strangers turned to smile an encouraging welcome as we made our way to our seats, and there were Joy and Derek with their children, all waving madly, delighted to see us.

The meeting started with a bang, just as the Celebration Evenings had done, with everybody singing and dancing about, waving their arms in the air and looking as if they were really enjoying themselves. No hushed tones and echoing vaulted roof here, but an atmosphere charged with anticipation. Anticipation of what? We had no idea, but the feeling was contagious.

I felt I belonged now. No longer was I an observer watching other people praising God; something had happened inside me and *I* wanted to praise him, too.

What a contrast to the last time we'd been here, at the carol service just before Christmas, when I had collapsed across Peter's lap in a state of exhaustion, my back and neck aching and my head thumping! Today, though I was still weak, I could think and speak clearly, the depression and pain were gone and for the first time in three years I was actually enjoying life.

'If you want us to pray with you,' announced the man who was leading the meeting, 'come out to the front here. Come right up to the platform.'

Peter was on his feet in a flash. I was amazed. Without a moment's hesitation he grabbed my hand and rushed me down the aisle to the front of the hall and up on the platform.

'Thank you, God,' he wept, tears of gratitude pouring down his face. 'Thank you for healing my wife.'

I knew now why Liz and Joy had stared at me when I was praying, for the most astonishing transformation was taking place in Peter right before my eyes. As he prayed his prayer of thanks to God, the same peace and joy and love which had filled me swept over him. I could see the burden of grief rolling from him, and that grin which seems to characterise all newly born-again Christians split his face from ear to ear.

Suddenly, Joy and Derek were beside us, hugging us, jubilation written all over their faces. As I turned to greet them I saw that the entire congregation were on their knees, thanking God. Then quietness swept over the room as the immensity of what God had done filled everyone with awe. We whispered our thanks to him, so wrapped up in our praying that the meeting finished half an hour later than usual.

'You do realise that we are the cause of everyone in Northgate Church having a burnt Sunday lunch?' said Peter, with mock severity. We were on our way home, after the meeting had finally ended, battered and exhausted from all the enthusiastic hugging. We laughed and sniggered like schoolchildren, driving along in silence for a few minutes, then catching one another's eye and snorting with laughter all over again.

Sally was quite confused by this startling change in her usually sober parents. For three years she had known nothing but doom and gloom, illness and depression. She had long denied the existence of God, but now she couldn't argue. The proof of what he could do was right before her eyes.

It took some time for the reality of our transformation finally to sink in for her, but as soon as she felt secure that it was a permanent state, that I really was healed, she too gave her life to God and had that same wonderful experience.

On Tuesday, I gathered up my basket of prepared food and went along as usual to the Psychiatric Unit for the day. As I pushed open the big glass doors I almost trod on Grace, who was standing just behind them. She was the girl with anorexia and religious mania who had seen me in my worst state after my overdose.

Her jaw dropped open when she saw me. 'Whatever's happened to you?' she asked, staring at me wide-eyed.

It was my turn to be startled. 'What's the matter?' I asked, wondering what she was looking at.

'You look better,' she said. 'You look totally different.'

'Well, I've been healed,' I replied. 'God healed me.'

'It *must* have been God,' she declared. 'Nothing else could change you like this.' Then she drifted up the corridor towards the ward as it was pill time.

I must admit I felt a bit shaken by her reaction. I knew how I felt inside, but was it really so obvious to other people? I stepped into the hall where Dr Johnstone's reception nurse, Betty, sat at her desk.

'Chris, whatever's happened?' she cried. 'You look completely different.'

'I've been healed,' I repeated. 'I'm better! I'm so happy now.'

'You wait there,' she commanded. 'Dr Johnstone has got to see this!' And she rushed off to arrange for him to see me in the middle of his busy outpatients' clinic while I wandered into the ward and made myself a drink. One by one the patients approached the table where I sat drinking my herbal tea.

'Is it really you, Chris?' they asked in disbelief. Some enquired wistfully, 'Tell us what happened. However did you do it?'

Nurses peeped through the window of the sister's office, their voices carrying through to the lounge where I waited. 'Have you seen Chris Youngman? She's sitting at the lounge table. Go and have a look at her.' Then Betty hurried in to tell me that Dr Johnstone was ready to see me.

I went round the corner into the corridor and saw Dr Johnstone, who had left his desk and was standing outside his room. He took one look at me and called in a loud voice, 'Chris! Come in here!'

I flung myself down the short hallway to reach him. Never before had he spoken to me like that; he was always gentle and supportive—and he had always called me Christine. But inside the tiny office his voice rang with exuberance.

'You look wonderful,' he said. 'I'm so thrilled for you. We've struggled for years but I've never really been able to help you.'

'You *have* helped me,' I insisted. 'You have!'

I loved this kind man with all my heart; he had been a lifeline of support to me throughout those difficult years.

'Make an appointment to see me at the earliest opportunity,' he said, and hurried back into his clinic.

I walked slowly out of the ward and into the day hospital and told the nurses there what had happened.

'Lovely, dear,' they said, smiling benevolently. 'Yes, you do look much better.' They weren't excited like the nurses in the ward, but I didn't care.

I stood for a moment, wondering what to do, where to go. Patients were all around me. Some were old friends, long-term people like myself, and others were newcomers whom I hadn't yet got to know. But all had one thing in common: they looked disturbed.

Some sat in the corner, as I had done so often, with

head bowed, mopping up the tears which flowed continually. Others were on their way to therapy groups. Many were sitting in the hallway, staring blankly or babbling mindlessly to themselves. I was supposed to spend the whole day at the unit but I realised, looking around, that I didn't belong here anymore. The thought of joining these people was horrific.

I turned and walked out through the glass double doors without looking back. As they swung shut behind me a great bubble of joy welled up inside as I realised I was free at last.

Three long years had passed since we as a family had first set out for that holiday in France. From being the happy, relaxing time we had looked forward to it had turned into a holiday in hell—a hell from which we had lost all hope of ever escaping.

But now I was back. The nightmare had ended—the shipwrecked sailor had finally reached the shore. My holiday in hell was over.

15

Food, glorious food!

I felt a bit of a fraud going back to stay at Joy's house, but I was still as weak as a kitten and quite incapable of doing housework. So, as Joy was eager to have me, I went along for a few days.

We sat down for tea and everyone started teasing me about my plate of boiled, mushy peas.

'It makes me feel sick,' said Derek with disgust. 'It puts me off my own food to see you having to eat that!'

'He prayed for you when he heard you were coming to stay again,' laughed Joy. ' *"Oh Lord, please save her from the green slime!"* '

Everyone was laughing, but after three years I'd come to accept my diet. I couldn't even remember what it was like to eat normally.

The next day, while Joy was baking in the kitchen, I took out my dowsing needle and began to test my food before preparing it for tea.

I had used the little needle ever since the evening we had spent at Joan's house when she had first introduced me to the practice. It had been faithfully accurate at first but, lately, it hadn't been totally reliable.

I was still using it in exactly the same way but, incredible as it sounds, there were times when I almost felt it had deliberately lied to me. I could never be absolutely sure that if I ate the foods the needle indicated, I would be all right. Most of the time I was, but occasionally I reacted badly and became ill.

'You shouldn't use that dowsing needle, Chris,' said Joy, looking up from what she was doing. 'It doesn't please God.'

'What do you mean?' I asked indignantly. 'Why should God object to it?'

'You've given your life to him now,' she insisted. 'Putting your trust in that thing means you're not trusting him to take care of you.'

I felt like exploding! I believed that using the needle to choose my food had saved my life. Why should I have to stop now?

Then I was suddenly aware of what God had done for me. I was well again, free from the Psychiatric Unit for ever. Joy was right. I could trust God to take care of me now. My anger drained away as I plucked the needle from my purse, walked across the room and threw it into the bin under the kitchen sink.

Joy looked shocked. 'You only did that to please me, didn't you?' she said sharply.

'No, I don't want it. I'm not going to use it anymore,' I declared. And I meant it.

That night, I went to bed dreaming of cornflakes and milk. The thought of eating a great bowl of them dominated my mind, and it was the first thing I thought of when I woke up the next morning.

'I'm going to have cornflakes and milk for breakfast,'

I announced when I got up. 'A whole bowlful.'

Joy was on the edge of panic. Milk was the very worst thing I could have—I was more allergic to that than anything else.

'If you're going to try drinking milk, don't you think you'd be better with just a drop in a cup of tea?' she suggested nervously. But I was determined.

The milky cereal tasted terrible! It was so long since I had eaten anything so rich that it felt like clots of fatty curds in my mouth. But I forced it down until I had eaten the lot.

Five minutes went by before the effect hit me. Then my head was exploding and my stomach burning, and panic tore through me as I reeled across the room and lurched into the radiator.

'Help me, God!' I cried in desperation. 'Take it away! Help me!'

And it just stopped. All was peace once again. I slumped down on a chair beside Joy at the kitchen table and we sat for a while, stunned by the miracle we had just witnessed.

On Saturday, the monthly Celebration Evening was held at Northgate Church. The room was crowded and very noisy with everybody leaping about in the aisles, shouting and singing as usual. It was going full swing when the guest speaker, Ron Tempest, held up his hand and stopped the musicians.

'God has told me there are many sick people here,' he said. 'Stand up if you want us to pray for you. God is going to heal you tonight.'

About ten people rose to their feet, eager to be made well again.

'That's not enough,' declared Ron firmly. 'God is telling me that there are many more. Musicians, play again for us. Let's give time for the others to take courage and stand up.'

We sang once more and by the end of the song about ten more people were on their feet.

Even then Ron wasn't satisfied. 'That's still not enough,' he persisted. 'God wants to help you. Please stand up so we can pray for you.'

I was praying for God to heal all the poor psychiatric patients I had left behind on the ward, when suddenly I thought, 'You fool! He wants to heal *you!*' Here I was, praying for everyone else, yet I was still so allergic to food that I was struggling to survive on practically nothing!

Up to that point, the thought of asking God specifically to heal my allergies had never crossed my mind—it was beyond my wildest dreams even to think of eating normally again. I was so grateful for feeling well that it hadn't occurred to me to ask for more.

In the middle of all the singing I stood up and shouted at the top of my voice, 'Oh, God, please heal my allergies!' I stayed on my feet until the song had ended, then Ron looked around the hall at the thirty people who were now standing, waiting for prayer.

'That's about it,' he declared. 'Now come forward and we'll pray for you.'

There were so many of us that the church elders prayed for us *en masse,* rather than individually. Then, exhausted by the effort, I made my way back to my seat and lay across Peter's knee.

The half-term holidays were upon us and we had made plans to visit friends in Yorkshire. I had already written to Linda and Tom, giving them a list of foods I could eat and which days I had to eat them, and telling Linda I would probably bring most of it with me.

The cookery basket sat on the work surface in the kitchen, piled high with nuts and the grain scones I'd made, with the water-filter beside it. I began collecting together the pills, drops and injections I would need to take with me when a quiet voice said, 'You don't need those.'

I looked up to see who had spoken, but no-one was there. I was completely alone in the room yet I had distinctly heard a voice speak to me. Could it be God speaking?

But what would happen if I stopped taking the pills which stopped my own body yeast from attacking me? What about the dreadful withdrawal effects from the psychiatric drugs? I knew from previous experience that just attempting to reduce the dose caused me to shake and drop things, leaving me trembling from head to foot.

And what about the cocktail of allergens which Dr King had made up specially for me? I couldn't get that anywhere else. The hospital sister had already warned me about trying to reduce the drug dosage without supervision—yet I was considering stopping it instantly! Years of medical training urged me not to risk it.

Torn by indecision, I put the drugs into the basket. Then

I took them out again and put them back into the cupboard. Then back in the basket . . . then into the cupboard.

I shut the cupboard door with a bang.

'If I'm healed, I don't need them,' I decided.

I hurried out to the car before I could change my mind, and we drove off. It was the craziest thing I had ever done, but I felt totally at peace about it.

It was late evening when we finally arrived at the remote village of Danby Whiske. A blizzard was blowing as we made our way down the narrow lanes to the old manor house where Tom and Linda lived.

Linda was cooking spaghetti bolognese and I joined her in the kitchen to prepare my crushed-pea scone. The bolognese smelt wonderful! I looked from my dry, grey little scone to the delicious savoury meat sauce and suddenly knew that I could safely try some. I wouldn't eat the spaghetti, just the sauce.

It was delicious and I suffered no ill effects at all.

Day by day I became more adventurous. Somehow, I would know quite clearly what to eat and what to avoid until, after two weeks, I found I could eat anything at all. The expected withdrawal symptoms from the drugs never materialised so, after a little while, I just forgot about them.

It was just the same when we went home after the holiday. Peter threw all my drugs away and I began to use my chlorine filter jug for watering the plants! I revelled greedily in eating chocolate, beefburgers and other junk food.

On Tuesday I had an appointment to see Dr Johnstone. He sat in his consulting room with my bulky case-sheets on his desk, observing me professionally, assessing whether or not my healing was genuine.

'To what do you actually ascribe this recovery?' he asked.

I felt embarrassed. After all, for the last two years he had done everything he could to help me and it had had little or no effect.

'I'm terribly sorry, Dr Johnstone, but it just has to be God,' I said.

'Don't apologise,' he replied gently. 'I'm just so pleased that you're feeling better—it doesn't matter how it happened.'

He sat for a few moments staring down at the file crammed with case-sheets about my long illness. 'I don't think I need to see you again, do I?' he decided.

For a second I felt frantic at the thought of losing his support. Only a month ago he had told Peter I would never recover, and they had talked about plans for my care. Now he was ready to discharge me. But the panic was soon over and I smiled at him.

'You've got so many sick people who need you,' I said. 'I'll be one less for you to look after.'

I watched as he wrote *Discharged* on my notes and closed the fat file for the last time.

The very next day Peter took me to Liverpool for our appointment with Dr King. We had to wait a long time before going in to see him but it was worth it to observe his face. He was amazed at the difference in me.

'What! Eaten *everything?*' he cried in disbelief. 'Are you seeing these church people again?'

'Of course we are,' Peter replied. 'We're very grateful. We go to the church every week now.'

'I should continue to do so,' advised the doctor. 'I've never been able to help you, Chris, but it appears that they have! I'm most interested in what's happened to you. Will you come back in six months' time and let me see how you've got on?'

When we did go back to see him six months later we found there was no waiting this time; we were ushered into his office as soon as we arrived.

'I'm delighted to see how well you are,' he said enthusiastically, as we eagerly told him I was gaining in strength every day. We rejoiced together, said goodbye, and closed another set of case-notes for the last time.

16

Something to shout about

'This lady has been healed of depression which lasted for almost three years, and allergies so severe they prevented her from living a normal life,' announced Bryn Jones to the thousands of people gathered in Leicester for the 'Day of God's Power' meeting.

'And what's more,' he went on, 'she's asked God to heal her muscles which wasted away so badly during her illness. And God is going to do it!'

'That's right!' roared the congregation. 'Hallelujah! God's going to do it!'

People from all over the north of England had come together for that Saturday in March. During the afternoon meeting, those who wanted God to heal them were encouraged to put their own hands on the part of their body which was painful or diseased. I couldn't make up my mind what to do as my entire body was so wasted, but eventually I placed my hands in the centre of my spine.

Nothing seemed to happen at the time but after the miracles I had experienced over the last four weeks I felt totally confident that God would act on my behalf.

Then suddenly, as I sat among the worshipping congregation, my back jolted upright with a bang! It gave me a terrible fright. Then I realised I was sitting completely upright for the first time in years. I stood up, my head held high with ease. And when I raised my arms in praise to God they shot into the air effortlessly—and they stayed up instead of flopping down!

Wild with excitement, I shouted praise and thanks to God at the top of my voice. All around me people were dancing, even up in the balconies. As I watched, I could see the upper floor bouncing up and down! It looked as if the whole thing would come crashing down around our ears, but the meeting ended in triumph with the building still standing.

From that day on I could walk straight and tall and my head never hung forward out of control again. Only a week later I was walking gracefully along a fashion show catwalk, modelling sweaters before a crowd of onlookers and photographers.

My knitting business, despite my illness, had continued to thrive and, since many of my original creations were being shown that night, I was there behind the scenes. But when it became obvious, as the evening went on, that the number of sweaters far exceeded the number of models, the organiser threw a massive cardigan over my shoulders and pushed me out on to the catwalk.

'Hey, I'm not a model!' I protested in alarm.

'Get on with it,' she hissed desperately from the wings.

With head held high and shoulders back I swung boldly down the catwalk performing a sort of rumba to the music, stopping to pose for the cameras, showing back and front views.

There were other triumphs, too. I knew that I had regained my rightful role as mother to Sally when the time came for her interview at the college of art. Her schooldays were coming to an end and, as she showed her folio of beautiful artwork, we knew the only thing that could stop her doing the job she really wanted was her lack of educational qualifications—which had suffered through the trauma of coping with my illness.

We sat together silently, awaiting the interviewers' verdict. Then, victory! She was accepted. We drove to our favourite little cafe to celebrate.

'I feel this is a turning point for me, Mum,' she confided. 'I always felt so sad when you were ill. Now I've got my whole future before me.'

But what was my own future to be? I felt well but I was still too weak to work. I couldn't walk very far and was still claiming invalidity benefit to finance the running of my car. But I began to feel uneasy about that. If I was essentially healed, how could I claim to be an invalid?

Common sense told me to wait until I was strong and well before giving up my allowance, but every time I told anyone I had been healed, that invalidity benefit haunted me, calling me a liar. It was time to act.

Dear Sir, I wrote. *I have been healed by Jesus at a meeting of God's Power and no longer need my invalidity benefit. I enclose my payment book and a poster advertising our meetings. Yours sincerely, Christine Youngman.*

The deed done, I dropped the letter in the post-box and

walked home without a care in the world.

Monday night saw the first Northgate Church ladies 'Pray and Weigh' meeting. All those who needed to shed a few pounds were coming together to discuss diets and encourage one another in fighting the flab. Now this was something I could help with. I offered to go along and supervise some keep-fit exercises.

'You can't come,' they protested. 'You're far too skinny. You'll show us all up!'

'Look, praying about losing weight is good,' I said, 'but a bit of exercise can only help speed up the process.' They agreed, and gratefully accepted my offer of help.

I took along some spare leotards for them to borrow and tapes of appropriate music. My own leotard hung like a sack on me as I stood at the front and hesitantly started to show them a warming-up exercise. Then I put the music on and watched them swing into action.

An incredible thing began to happen to me as I stood there. Power surged through me, strengthening my muscles as my body came to life. I leapt to the music, dancing, kicking, joining in the whole routine. Everyone stared at the amazing sight. One of the girls wept as she realised the significance of what was happening before her eyes.

I had only come along with the intention of supervising the class but here I was, leading the way. I was a keep-fit teacher again! Week by week the girls got thinner and I got fatter as my muscles grew. Joy wept with wonder at the sight of me. She and Derek invited us out for dinner at a restaurant to celebrate. 'And none of your green slime, either,' he teased. 'We're going to have a *proper* meal.'

News of my remarkable recovery swept through the town as reporters came to interview me for their newspapers. 'LIFE IS LOOKING LOVELY FOR CHRIS' declared the headlines in the local paper.

It wasn't long before the national dailies got hold of the story. 'DOCTORS BAFFLED BY MUM'S MIRACLE' announced the *Sunday People,* while *Weekend* magazine described me as 'MOTHER COURAGE', showing photographs of me jogging and riding my bike.

'I'm baffled by Mrs Youngman's rapid recovery,' confessed Dr King, the allergy specialist, when reporters interviewed him. 'She was in a very bad way and I wouldn't have expected her to get better for many years, if at all.'

Week by week I grew stronger, gradually taking on all my own housework, teaching keep-fit classes, playing the piano three times a week in a cafe and painting pictures to sell.

I never did return to my beloved Rehabilitation Unit. While I was ill it was demolished and the work transferred to a smart new hospital.

But somehow it didn't matter, because my priorities had changed. Nor did I pursue the art therapy course. It was a career for a disabled person, and I had thoroughly recovered now.

Two years went by and those who had shaken their heads in disbelief at my miraculous healing began to realise that it was a permanant state, not a nine-day wonder.

Dales Television, a Christian television company,

approached us, asking permission to make a video of my story. They arrived with a van-load of equipment and set about filming us in and around our home. Family, friends and former colleagues were interviewed before the cameras and all gave testimony to the desperate state I'd been in and the astonishing difference in me.

Dr Billington consented to be interviewed in his consulting room, so the producer, Julian Boden, turned up with all his equipment, his sound technician and his camera operator and somehow they squashed themselves into the tiny room at the surgery.

'What condition was Chris in when you first saw her on her return from France?' he asked.

'She was very weak and lethargic,' replied the doctor. 'Her hands and feet were very cold and even short walks made her quite exhausted.

'When she didn't pick up she became progressively more and more depressed at her lack of progress,' he went on. 'She was incapable of coping with work or running her home.'

He explained my food allergies and the different treatments they had tried to curb the relentless progress of the disease.

'Observing Chris's deterioration over the years, what were your feelings about her future?' Julian wondered.

'I was quite disturbed about the future,' Dr Billington replied. 'It was difficult to see the way ahead. We felt from our point of view that we'd tried all we could and hadn't made a lot of progress.'

'So when you see Chris now, how fit do you think

she is?'

'She's amazingly fit!' answered Dr Billington with conviction. 'She's a very active person, running the house, holding down a job and teaching a keep-fit class. She made a very dramatic recovery.'

The video film was released as part of a series, under the title *They Claim a Miracle—The Chris Youngman Story.* It has been shown all over the country in churches, schools and private homes, telling of the power of God to heal, not just in Bible days but now, in this twentieth century.

Several years have passed since that day when God changed my life in Joy's front room, and I'm still as fit as ever.

Many people ask why God chose to heal me when so many other people continue to be sick. I honestly don't know. But I have learned through my illness to identify with sick friends.

I have found, too, that I love people far more now than I did even in my days as a physio. *I've been there—I know how they feel.* I can let them know that God loves each one of them as individuals, whether ill or well. Yes, getting to know him personally has caused me to view life with new eyes!

And, of course, the dynamic of God's power has had lasting effects not only in my own life: he has reached into our family, changed each one of us individually, then bound us together in the security of his love.

From the chilling nightmare of a holiday in hell he caught us up into the warm sunshine of the joy of heaven.